Spinal Cord Injury

9-30-14   #19.95

DATE DUE			

AMERICAN ACADEMY OF NEUROLOGY (AAN)
Quality of Life Guides
Lisa M. Shulman, MD
Series Editor

Alzheimer's Disease
Paul Dash, MD and Nicole Villemarette-Pittman, PhD

Amyotrophic Lateral Sclerosis
Robert G. Miller, MD, Deborah Gelinas, MD, and Patricia O'Connor, RN

Epilepsy
Ilo E. Leppik, MD

Guillain-Barré Syndrome
Gareth John Parry, MB, ChB, FRACP and Joel Steinberg, MD, PhD

Migraine and Other Headaches
William B. Young, MD and Stephen D. Silberstein, MD

Peripheral Neuropathy
Norman Latov, MD

Restless Legs Syndrome
Mark J. Buchfuhrer, MD, Wayne A. Hening, MD, PhD,
and Clete Kushida, MD, PhD

Spinal Cord Injury
Michael E. Selzer, MD, PhD and Bruce H. Dobkin, MD

Stroke
Louis R. Caplan, MD

Understanding Pain
Harry J. Gould, III, MD, PhD

Spinal Cord Injury

MICHAEL E. SELZER, MD, PhD
Department of Neurology
University of Pennsylvania
and
Office of Research and Development
US Department of Veterans Affairs

BRUCE H. DOBKIN, MD
Department of Neurology
University of California at Los Angeles
and
Dr. Miriam and Sheldon G. Adelson
Medical Research Foundation

LISA M. SHULMAN, MD
Series Editor
Associate Professor of Neurology
Rosalyn Newman Distinguished Scholar in Parkinson's Disease
Co-Director, Maryland Parkinson's Disease
and Movement Disorders Center
University of Maryland School of Medicine
Baltimore, Maryland

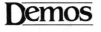
New York

A A N P R E S S
AMERICAN ACADEMY OF
NEUROLOGY

Demos Medical Publishing LLC, 386 Park Avenue South, New York, New York 10016

Library of Congress Cataloging-in-Publication Data
Spinal cord injury / Michael E. Selzer ... [et al.].
   p. cm.
Includes index.
ISBN-13: 978-1-932603-38-5 (pbk. : alk. paper)
ISBN-10: 1-932603-38-7 (pbk. : alk. paper)
1. Spinal cord—Wounds and injuries—Popular works. I. Selzer, Michael E.
RD594.3.S66528   2008
617.4'82044—dc22
                                     2008000444

Special discounts on bulk quantities of Demos Medical Publishing books are available to corporations, professional associations, pharmaceutical companies, health care organizations and other qualifying groups. For details, please contact:

Special Sales Department
Demos Medical Publishing
386 Park Avenue South, Suite 301
New York, NY 10016
Phone: (800) 532-8663; (212) 683-0072
Fax: 212-683-0118
Email ordering: orderdept@demosmedpub.com

Made in the United States of America
08 09 10   5 4 3 2 1

Contents

About the AAN Press Quality of Life Guides

IN THE SPIRIT OF THE DOCTOR-PATIENT PARTNERSHIP

THE BETTER-INFORMED PATIENT is often able to play a vital role in his or her own care. This is especially the case with neurologic disorders, for which effective management of disease can be promoted—indeed, *enhanced*—through patient education and involvement.

In the spirit of the partnership-in-care between physicians and patients, the American Academy of Neurology Press is pleased to produce a series of "Quality of Life" guides on an array of diseases and ailments that affect the brain and central nervous system. The series, produced in partnership with Demos Medical Publishing, answers a number of basic and important questions faced by patients and their families.

Additionally, the authors, most of whom are physicians and all of whom are experts in the areas in which they write, provide a detailed discussion of the disorder, its causes, and the course it may follow. You also find strategies for coping with the disorder and handling a number of nonmedical issues.

The result: As a reader, you will be able to develop a framework for understanding the disease and become better prepared to manage the life changes associated with it.

ABOUT THE AMERICAN ACADEMY OF NEUROLOGY (AAN)

The American Academy of Neurology is the premier organization for neurologists worldwide. In addition to support of educational and scientific advances, the AAN—along with its sister organization, the AAN Foundation—is a strong advocate of public education and a leading supporter of research for breakthroughs in neurologic patient care.

More information on the activities of the AAN is available on our website, www.aan.com. For a better understanding of common disorders of the brain, as well as to learn about people living with these disorders, please turn to the AAN Foundation's website, www.thebrainmatters.org.

About Neurology and Neurologists

Neurology is the medical specialty associated with disorders of the brain and central nervous system. Neurologists are medical doctors with specialized training in the diagnosis, treatment, and management of patients suffering from neurologic disease.

Lisa M. Shulman, MD
Series Editor
AAN Press Quality of Life Guides

Preface

S PINAL CORD INJURY (SCI) is a devastating disorder that is especially poignant because it so often occurs in young adults who are just entering their most productive work and family years. Once a virtual death sentence, SCI now is medically manageable and its victims survive many years, essentially living a normal lifespan. Yet SCI patients may have severe ongoing disabilities that require assistance from caregivers, most often family. And because their injury may leave them vulnerable to many medical complications, victims of SCI constantly must be vigilant and some require frequent clinical attention. This book is intended to help persons with SCI, their families, loved ones and caregivers better understand the scientific basis for the disabilities that result from SCI, the current medical treatments and rehabilitative management of SCI, and the research directions that point to hope for better functional recovery in the future. At the end of the book there is a glossary of terms. It includes not only words found in this book, but other words you are likely to run into when reading about SCI. There is also a list of internet sites where additional useful information can be found. With this information in hand, patients and their caregivers can make better decisions about their medical management.

Spinal Cord Injury

CHAPTER 1

How Does the Spinal Cord Work and What Happens When It Doesn't?

THE SPINAL CORD is an extremely vital part of the central nervous system, and even a small injury to it can lead to severe disability. For this reason, nature has encased the spinal cord within the thick layers of bone of the spinal column and surrounding muscle. Nevertheless, because it compresses so much function into such a narrow structure, the spinal cord is vulnerable to injury and disease.

People who have had a spinal cord injury can improve their ability to cope with their disabilities by learning about the functioning of a healthy spinal cord. The aim of this book is to help people with spinal cord injuries and their caregivers understand how the body responds when the spinal cord is injured, and how health care professionals approach the acute treatment and long-term management of the resulting disabilities.

More than 10,000 people in the United States are disabled by traumatic spinal cord injury (SCI) each year. The financial cost of these injuries can be enormous, depending on the severity and location of the

> More than 10,000 people in the United States are disabled by traumatic spinal cord injury (SCI) each year.

injury. Because of the medical advances that can keep these patients alive, approximately 230,000 people are currently living with traumatic

SCI in the U.S. Many more cases of SCI are caused by diseases such as tumors, infections, *amyotrophic lateral sclerosis* (ALS, or Lou Gehrig's disease), and multiple sclerosis.

NERVES: THE BUILDING BLOCKS OF THE NERVOUS SYSTEM

In order to understand the functioning of the spinal cord, the nervous system must be understood. The role of the nervous system is to receive information about the state of the body and its environment, to process that information in a way that permits a person to respond in a useful way, and generate command signals that cause the muscles, glands, and other organs to carry out desired actions, such as the movement of a limb or the release of a hormone.

The nerve cells (*neurons*) are the basic building blocks of the nervous system. Although nerve cells come in different sizes and shapes, and are made of different specialized chemical compositions, most neurons have a common basic structure consisting of three main parts:

- **Cell body, or *soma*.** The cell body contains the *nucleus*. This is where most of the chemicals necessary for functioning of the nerves are made.
- **Axon.** Nerve cells communicate with each other by generating an electrical signal that is transmitted over long distances along a cable-like structure called the *axon*.
- **Dendrites.** The *dendrites* are branches that arise from the cell body. They receive information from other nerve cells, which comes as electrical signals that either increase or decrease the excitability of the nerve cell. Information received by the dendrites is integrated into a common decision about whether to fire off a signal to other nerve cells. If the answer is "yes," an electrical signal is transmitted along the axon (Figure 1-1).

HOW AXONS AND DENDRITES COMMUNICATE

The axon has a swelling at its end called a *synaptic terminal*. This terminal is in close contact with a specialized area on the next neuron in the

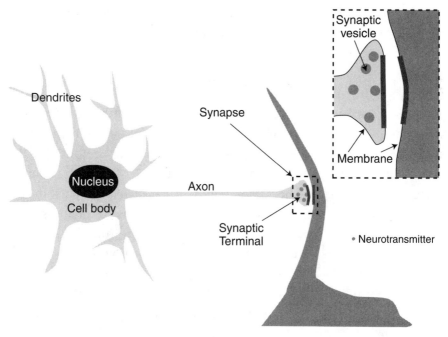

FIGURE 1-1

Neurons are the Basic Building Blocks of the Nervous System. This figure shows one neuron, in light gray, whose axon ends in a synaptic terminal filled with small vesicles of neurotransmitter (gray dots). The synaptic terminal is in close proximity to the dendrite of a second neuron (dark gray). When an electrical signal arrives at the synaptic terminal, the vesicles fuse with the presynaptic membrane, i.e., the part of the cell membrane surrounding the presynaptic terminal that is directly facing the postsynaptic dendrite and release neurotransmitters into the synaptic space. The pre- and post-synaptic membranes are thickened (dark lines in the inset enlargement) where they face each other across the synaptic space, where they are specialized to perform the communication function. The molecules of transmitter bind to receptor molecules on the post-synaptic membrane and produce a graded electrical signal in the post-synaptic neuron. In real life, the surfaces of cell bodies and dendrites receive thousands of synaptic terminals from many other neurons.

chain of communication, which is called the *post-synaptic membrane*. Each neuron in the central nervous system receives information from hundreds, or even thousands, of other neurons through *synapses* located along the dendrites and cell body. When the electrical signal reaches the *synaptic terminal*, a chemical called a *neurotransmitter* is released that either excites or inhibits the *post-synaptic membrane*. In this way, the post-

3

synaptic neuron is either more or less likely to fire an electrical signal to the next cell in the chain of communication (Figure 1-1).

STRUCTURE OF THE SPINAL CORD

The spinal cord is a long, tube-shaped structure that receives sensory information from the body via sensory neurons and transmits the information to the brain. Information is also relayed from the brain to the rest of the body via the motor neurons (Figure 1-2). The neck region of the spinal cord is called the *cervical* region. It has eight segments, meaning that it receives sensory information and transmits command signals to move muscles through eight sets of spinal nerves from the skin and muscles of the arms and neck. The chest is supplied by the twelve segments of the *thoracic* region of the spinal cord, and the legs are supplied by the five lumbar segments of the spinal cord and the first two of the five *sacral* segments. The buttocks and anus are supplied by the lowest three segments of the sacral spinal cord.

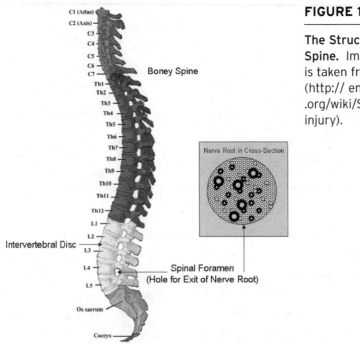

FIGURE 1-2

The Structure of the Spine. Image of spine is taken from Wikipedia (http:// en.wikipedia .org/wiki/Spinal_cord_ injury).

The nerves of the body merge as they approach the spinal cord to form the spinal nerves. Each major nerve has thousands of individual nerve fibers (*axons*), ranging in diameter from less than one-thousandth

> The spinal cord is a long, tube-shaped structure that receives sensory information from the body via sensory neurons and transmits the information to the brain. Information is also relayed from the brain to the rest of the body via the motor neurons.

of a millimeter to 20-thousandths of a millimeter. The larger the diameter of the axon, the faster it conducts electrical impulses. However, the larger the diameter of the axon, the more area its surface membrane has for electrical activity to leak where it should not go. This can slow electrical conduction, and also cause electrical activation of nearby nerve fibers that should not be active. In order to avoid this, large axons are insulated by a fatty material called myelin. The smallest diameter axons do not need *myelin*.

The spinal cord is contained within the spinal canal, which is inside the boney spine. The spine is composed of individual bones called *vertebrae*. Each vertebra is separated from the next by a cushion of fibrous, connective tissue called an *intervertebral disc*. The spinal cord stretches from the base of the skull to about 3 inches above the top of the hips; the boney spine extends to below the top of the hips, all the way to the middle of the buttocks. Thus, the boney spine and the spinal canal inside it are longer than the spinal cord itself. The spinal nerves of the lumbar and sacral levels must therefore span the distance from their exit level in the spinal cord to the level of the *spinal foramen* so they can leave the spine and distribute to the skin, muscles, and internal organs that they supply. The lower the spinal level, the longer this distance, and the longer the spinal nerve will travel in the spinal canal.

Because of its stringy appearance, the collection of lumbar and sacral nerves in the spinal canal below the level at which the spinal cord ends is called the *cauda equina*, which in Latin means "horse's tail." The end of the spinal cord contains the nerve cells of the sacral segments and is called the *conus medullaris*, which ends at about the level of the nerve root of the first lumbar vertebra (L1; see Figure 1-2).

The spinal cord has an inner core of gray matter containing neurons. Surrounding the gray matter is the white matter, which contains axons that carry messages between neurons at different levels of the spinal cord, and between the spinal cord and the brain. In medical language, the surfaces of body parts that face the back are called *dorsal*, and the surfaces facing the front are called *ventral*.

In Figure 1-3, the spinal cord is viewed in cross sections, as if to illustrate a person who is lying on her stomach with her head aimed at the upper right-hand corner. The neurons in the dorsal half of the gray matter serve sensory functions, and the neurons in the ventral half of the gray matter serve motor functions. These include the actual motor neurons, whose axons go to the muscles and cause them to contract. As the nerves approach the spinal cord they separate into two roots:

1. A dorsal root composed of sensory axons
2. A ventral root composed of motor axons

The neurons belonging to the dorsal root axons are located in the *dorsal root ganglion*, which is located outside the spinal cord. Sensory axons are able to transmit sensation because they make synapses with other nerve cells in the spinal cord or brain. Like the spinal cord itself, the dorsal root ganglion is contained within the boney spine.

The axons of the motor neurons leave the spinal cord by the ventral nerve roots, and continue in motor nerves to the muscles (Figure 1-4). Electrical impulses travel to the ends of the motor axons to reach the muscle cells, where they form large, complex synapses called *neuromuscular junctions*. There, the axons release a neurotransmitter called *acetylcholine*, which causes the muscle cells to become electrically excited and contract, thereby shortening the muscle. This, in turn, moves the parts of the body to which the muscle is attached. Sensory nerve endings in the muscles measure the degree of stretch, sending an electrical signal to the *motoneurons* in the spinal cord when the muscle is lengthened.

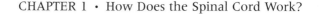

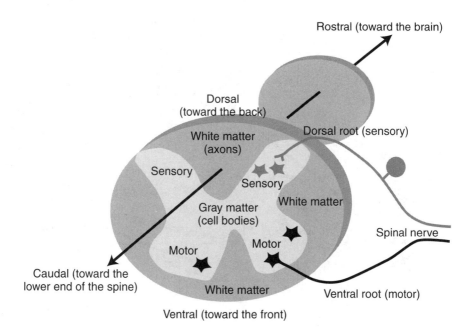

FIGURE 1-3

Organization of the Spinal Cord. The gray matter is a butterfly-shaped column of neural tissue on the inside of the spinal cord; it contains the neuron cell bodies. The white matter is on the outside. It contains the axons that run up and down the cord, connecting the different levels of the cord to each other and to the brain. The color of the white matter is due to the myelin insulation that surrounds the axons. Sensory information enters the spinal cord at each level via the dorsal roots. Motor output exits the spinal cord via the ventral roots. The cell bodies of sensory neurons are located in the dorsal root ganglia outside the spinal cord, but within the boney spine. The sensory and motor roots merge within the neural foramen as they leave the spinal canal to form the spinal nerve.

This sensory feedback causes the motoneurons to fire electrical impulses and activate the muscle. For example, this automatic response and can be seen when a doctor hits the tendon of the thigh muscle (*quadriceps*) just below the kneecap, stretching the thigh muscle. The subsequent twitching of the quadriceps muscle and kicking motion of the leg is called a *reflex*. Reflexes are the simplest forms of behavior.

Branches of the sensory axons that activate the motor neurons travel to the brainstem in the dorsal white matter. They provide the brain with information about the state of muscle contraction. Nerve cells in

7

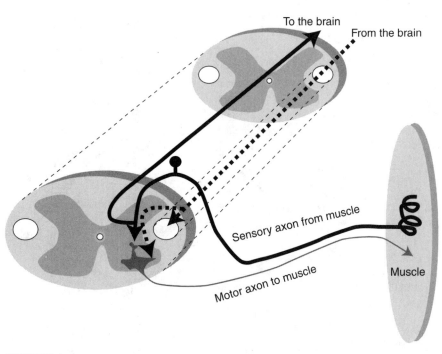

FIGURE 1-4

Spinal Cord Pathways that Control Muscles. Muscles are activated by axons coming from motor neurons in the spinal cord. These motor neurons can be activated by signals coming from the brain. The largest of these descending pathways is the corticospinal tract (thick dashed lines). Stretch of the muscle is detected by sensory nerve fibers (thick solid lines), which feed back a reflex activation of the motor neuron to cause a contraction of the stretched muscle. This protective mechanism prevents joints from suddenly being bent too far, but it also has other important uses in motor control.

the brain send axons to the spinal cord to instruct the motor neurons to initiate movements. The largest of these descending pathways from the brain, the *corticospinal tract*, is shown in white. Thus, the corticospinal pathway is part of the motor system. The axons of the corticospinal tract cross sides in the *medulla* (the lowest part of the brain), so that the left side of the brain controls the right side of the body and vice versa.

Sensations from the body reach the brain via axons ascending in two main pathways:

1. Large myelinated axons, carrying sensations of light touch, joint position, and vibration, ascend in the dorsal columns on the same

side as the dorsal root by which they enter the spinal cord. These fibers also transmit information that allows the brain to interpret, for example, how much a held object weighs and the fine details of its shape and texture. In other words, the dorsal columns carry high-resolution information about sensory stimuli.

2. Smaller axons carry a wide range of sensory modalities, including pain and temperature, which are not transmitted in the dorsal columns and are not carried directly to the brain. Instead these sensory fibers form synapses (connections) with second-order sensory neurons in the back part of the spinal cord gray matter (*dorsal horn*). These relay neurons send their axons across the midline of the spinal cord to the *anterolateral column* (also called the *anterior spinothalamic tract*) on the other side of the spinal cord.

From Figure 1-5, you can see that damage to the central part of the spinal cord can interrupt pain and temperature sensory information by damaging these secondary sensory nerve fibers. This becomes important when we consider the specific syndromes produced as a consequence of spinal cord injury.

Each muscle, internal organ, or patch of skin has a nerve that connects to a particular level of the spinal cord. Because of this, injuries to

> Damage to the central part of the spinal cord can interrupt pain and temperature sensory information by damaging the secondary sensory nerve fibers.

the spinal cord produce paralysis or loss of sensation in specific patterns. Knowing which muscles are paralyzed, or where in the body sensation has been lost, allows the examining doctor to determine with high accuracy where in the spinal cord the injury is located.

An important principle of organization in the spinal cord is that axons in both the corticospinal pathway, which carries motor commands from the brain to the spinal cord, and the anterior spinothalamic pathway, which carries sensory information from the spinal cord to the brain, are

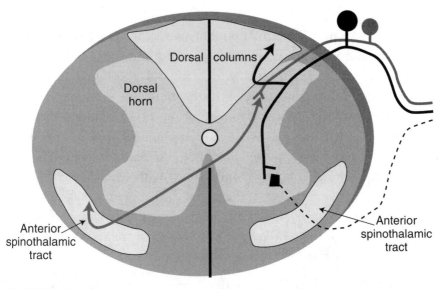

FIGURE 1-5

Spinal Cord Pathways that Mediate Sensation. The sensory pathways are organized so that the largest axons, which transmit sensations of vibration, joint position, sense and fine touch discrimination, and the ability to estimate the weight of an object, are carried in the dorsal column on the same side of the spinal cord as the dorsal root through which they enter (black). The dorsal columns also receive a branch of the nerve fibers that carry information about how much a muscle is stretched. These fibers send a branch (black) into the ventral horn of the spinal cord to activate the motor neurons that supply the same muscle. Temperature and pain sensations are not carried in the dorsal columns. Instead, axons carrying these sensations (gray) form relays in the dorsal horn with second order sensory neurons, whose axons cross to the other side of the spinal cord and travel in the anterolateral column (the anterior spinothalamic tract) to the brain.

organized so that nerve fibers from a given level of the spinal cord travel together. The lowest parts of the body are represented by the outermost fibers of the anterior spinothalamic or corticospinal tract. The highest parts of the body are represented by the innermost fibers (Figure 1-6).

How the Spinal Cord Works

The spinal cord is well protected by the boney spine (Figure 1-2). Yet, for reasons that are only partially understood, even injuries that fail to pen-

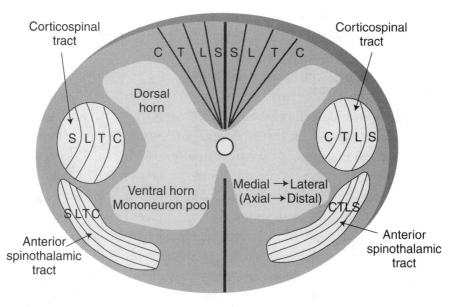

FIGURE 1-6

Segmental Organization of the Spinal Cord. The spinal cord is organized in a regular way, which influences how injuries produce neurological dysfunction. At any spinal cord level, the motor neurons of the ventral horn are placed so that those supplying the muscles of the trunk are innermost and those supplying the muscles furthest from the trunk, e.g., the fingers or toes, outermost. At any spinal cord level, the corticospinal and anterior spinothalamic tracts are organized so that the fibers that represent the parts of the body closest to that spinal level are innermost, and those that represent the lowest (most sacral) parts of the body are located outermost. However, the dorsal columns are organized with the highest parts of the body represented outermost, and the lowest parts of the body represented innermost. *C*, cervical; *T*, thoracic; *L*, lumbar; *S*, sacral.

etrate the spine can result in severe spinal cord damage and devastating paralysis through a vicious cycle called the *ischemic cascade*. What is clear is that concussion of the spinal cord—for example, an indirect injury from a blow to the spine that causes the spinal cord to bump into the inside surface of the spinal canal—causes a choking off of the internal blood flow in the center of the spinal cord.

Insufficient blood flow is called *ischemia*. In SCI, it can affect the cells of the spinal cord and the capillaries, causing them to leak. This results in *edema*, an abnormal accumulation of fluid that causes the spinal cord to swell. In addition, ischemic cells absorb too much calcium from the surrounding fluid and calcium-dependent biochemical reactions in the cells, leading to damaged membranes.

Certain genes can create "cell suicide" (*apoptosis*), activating biochemical pathways that break up the genetic material (DNA) into small pieces and cause the cell to break up into neat packets that are easily disposed of (see Chapter 8). Partially-damaged neurons become abnormally activated and release the excitatory neurotransmitter *glutamate*, which binds to receptors that open the cell membrane to more calcium entry. Ischemia impairs the ability of cells to re-accumulate the released glutamate, which, in turn, causes more nerve cell death by a process called *excitotoxicity*. The presence of injured and dead cells invites white blood cells to release chemicals called *cytokines*, resulting in inflammation.

Some of these cytokines are injurious to neurons; they make the white blood cells more effective at attacking damaged nerve cells; and they cause more edema. This produces further swelling and cell death in a vicious cycle, resulting in delayed damage (*secondary neuronal damage*). No anatomic abnormality can be seen during the first 8 hours or so after an impact injury. But as time passes, small hemorrhages appear in the center of the spinal cord, spreading outward and leaving a rim of white matter (axons) in the outer layers of the spinal cord.

No one knows why the spinal cord is so exquisitely sensitive to concussive injury, but because the spinal canal is only 50 percent wider than the spinal cord, when swelling causes the diameter of the cord to increase by 50 percent, it is compressed against the inner surface of the spinal canal, causing even more tissue damage. This is a vicious cycle, indeed.

SYMPTOMS OF SPINAL CORD INJURY

The symptoms of SCI depend on the severity and level of the injury.

Because the bladder and bowel are controlled by the sacral spinal segments low in the spinal cord, complete injury at almost any level will impair control of urination and defecation. Similarly, SCI at the lumbar or thoracic levels will cause paralysis and loss of sensation of the legs, but not the arms.

Injury in the low cervical region will cause weakness or paralysis in the hands, but the arms and shoulder will have strength. Respiration will be spared enough to breathe without a respirator because the diaphragm is controlled by the upper cervical segments. However,

> The symptoms of SCI depend on the severity and level of the injury.

because the muscles of the rib cage participate in respiration and are innervated by thoracic segments, breathing will be weaker than normal in all patients with cervical SCI, and their endurance will be limited. Moreover, the ability to cough will be limited, causing difficulty clearing the airway of saliva and nasal secretions.

Injury in the mid-cervical region will cause paralysis and numbness of the arms, hands, and legs, but the muscles of the shoulder and neck will be spared. High cervical injuries will cause paralysis and numbness of the entire body below the neck, and will also impair breathing, often requiring a respirator to maintain life.

Blood pressure is controlled to a great degree by a specialized part of the nervous system called the *sympathetic nervous system*. Because the nerve supply from the spinal cord to the *sympathetic ganglia* arises in the thoracic and lumbar spinal cord segments, cervical spinal cord injuries separate the sympathetic outflow from areas in the brain that are responsible for modulating that outflow, causing the blood pressure to be unstable because of exaggerated local sympathetic reflexes. This can lead to severe headaches when the blood pressure undergoes wide swings from low to high. The specific neurologic deficits associated with injuries at different spinal cord levels are summarized in the Table 1-1.

Spasticity

A feature of the weakness seen in SCI is that the muscles become stiff. This is the opposite of how muscles respond to loss of innervation by motor neurons, which is to become limp. The spinal cord has neural cir-

Table 1-1 Neurologic Deficits of People with SCI at Different Levels

Spinal Level	Neurologic Defects
C1-C3	Loss of breathing control–ventilator dependent; inability to clear saliva from throat by coughing; inability to speak, but might be able to communicate with a mouth stick and computer because neck flexion, extension, and rotation are preserved; loss of bowel and bladder control; paralysis of arms, hands, trunk, and legs; unable to shift in bed; needs 24-hour-a-day care.
C4	May be able to breathe, but often needs some ventilator assistance; loss of bowel and bladder control, weak speech–may need mouth stick and computer to communicate; paralysis of arms, hands, trunk, and legs, unable to shift in bed; needs 24-hour-a-day care.
C5	Able to use diaphragm, but breathing is weak because of paralysis of chest muscles (intercostal muscles between the ribs)–low endurance; weak cough–may need help clearing saliva; can speak; loss of bowel and bladder control; can move shoulders and flex elbows, but cannot extend arms at elbows; paralysis of wrists, hands, trunk, and legs; can relieve pressure by moving in bed with help of some equipment; cannot get out of bed without assistance; needs help sitting up for eating, but then can eat using special utensils; can use a power-assisted wheelchair and might be able to use a manual wheelchair indoors. Needs 6 hours of assistance per day for personal care, and 10 hours per day for home care.
C6	Able to use diaphragm, but breathing is weak because of paralysis of chest muscles–low endurance; weak cough–may need help clearing saliva; can speak; loss of bowel and bladder control, but might be able to manipulate waste-collection bags and other adaptive devices; can move shoulders and flex elbows, but cannot extend arms at elbows; paralysis of wrist flexion, but can extend the wrist (bend it back); paralysis of hands, trunk, and legs; can relieve pressure by moving in bed and wheelchair with help of some equipment; can use adaptive eating utensils except for knife; needs some help to get out of bed; can use a power-assisted or manual wheelchair, but needs help with manual wheelchair outdoors. Needs 6 hours of assistance per day for personal care, and 4 hours per day for home care.
C7-C8	Able to use diaphragm, but breathing is weak because of paralysis of chest muscles–low endurance; weak cough–may need help clearing saliva; can speak; loss of bowel and bladder control; can move shoulders, arms, wrists, and hands; paralysis of trunk and legs; can relieve pressure by moving in bed or wheelchair; most can get in and out of bed or wheelchair without help; can eat independently, although some adaptive devices are helpful; can stand, although might need

Spinal Level	Neurologic Defects
	some help; cannot walk; can use a power-assisted wheelchair anywhere, and a manual wheelchair indoors, but might need help with uneven terrain outdoors; can drive an adapted car. Needs 6 hours of assistance per day for personal care, and 2 hours per day for home care.
T1–T9	Breathing slightly weak and endurance less than normal; although there is no voluntary control of the bowel and bladder, able to take care of bowel and bladder hygiene using intermittent catheterization, bowel suppositories, and other techniques; can move shoulders, arms, wrists, and hands; paralysis of lower trunk and legs; can get in and out of bed or wheelchair without help; can eat independently; can stand with a standing frame (similar to a walker, but with a seat that tilts to give variable support and help shift from sitting to standing), but cannot walk; can use a manual wheelchair independently; can drive a hand-controlled car. Needs no assistance for personal care, and only 3 hours per day for heavy work in housekeeping.
T10–L1	Normal breathing and endurance; able to take care of bowel and bladder; good trunk stability, but legs paralyzed; can get in and out of bed or wheelchair without help; can stand and walk with forearm crutches or walker, wearing a knee-ankle-foot orthosis (KAFO); can use a manual wheelchair independently; can drive a hand-controlled car. Needs no assistance for personal care, and only 2 hours per day for heavy work in housekeeping.
L2–S5	Normal breathing and endurance; able to take care of bowel and bladder; good trunk stability, and some strength in legs; can get in and out of bed or wheelchair without help; can stand and walk with forearm crutches or cane, wearing a knee-ankle-foot orthosis or ankle-foot orthosis; can use a manual wheelchair independently; can drive a hand-controlled car. Needs no assistance for personal care, and 0-1 hour per day for heavy work in housekeeping.

cuitry, which assures an ongoing amount of muscle tone by keeping the motor neurons active. The muscles have sensory nerve fibers that send signals to the spinal cord whenever a muscle is subjected to stretching. This signal causes a reflexive contraction of the same muscle to protect it from overstretching, and to assure that the limbs remain in a useful posture.

For example, the quadriceps muscles of the thigh insert into the lower leg by the *patellar tendon*, which goes over the knee cap (*patella*). If a person jumps up and lands on their feet, the weight of the body would ordinarily cause the knee to buckle. However, the buckling would sub-ject the quadriceps muscles to sudden stretching, which would result in a corrective reflex contraction of the quadriceps muscles and straighten-ing of the legs. If there were no reflex-damping mechanism, the sensory signals from each muscle to the spinal cord might keep all of the muscles in a constant state of excessive tension, and a person would be frozen in place, unable to move. Moreover, because each contraction of one mus-cle results in the stretching of an opposing muscle, unrestrained muscle stretch reflexes prevent any movement from occurring.

Fortunately, in an uninjured person, the brain exerts an ongoing inhibition of these muscle stretch reflexes and keeps the muscles loose. When the brain sends a message via the spinal cord to move a limb, it also removes the inhibition to the motor neurons controlling just the muscles involved, while maintaining or increasing the inhibition of opposing muscles. This allows the necessary contraction to occur.

In people with SCI, the ongoing inhibitory signals from the brain are removed from the spinal cord segments below the injury, which keeps the muscles in a constant state of tension. The exaggerated stretch reflexes can also be demonstrated when they are tested with a reflex hammer. For example, when the patellar tendon connecting the quadri-ceps muscles to the shin bone (*femur*) is struck with a hammer just below the knee cap, the resulting stretch of the quadriceps muscles caus-es a reflex contraction, which results in a kicking motion. In people with spinal cord injury, this type of kicking motion is abnormally violent.

Spasticity results from the interruption of the corticospinal pathway from the brain to the spinal cord, and the combination of increased mus-cle tone and exaggerated muscle stretch reflexes. In the legs, spasticity tends to affect the extensor muscles, which are the muscles that straight-en the legs and point the toes down, more than the flexors, which are the muscles that bend the legs and point the toes up. This is why people with SCI have their legs extended and might need help bending them to sit in a chair.

Paradoxically, in cases of incomplete SCI, spasticity in the legs can help support the person's weight when walking, so there might be advantages to it. However, because the muscles are not totally numb in these cases, the spasticity can give rise to painful cramps. Spasticity can be managed with physical therapy and medication.

GRADING THE SEVERITY OF SPINAL CORD INJURY

The nerves fibers that carry sensation to the spinal cord—and motor control impulses from the spinal cord to the muscles—are bundled together into large spinal nerves. Thus, the function of the spinal cord is mapped according to the functions represented in these main nerves. However, as they approach the spinal cord, the spinal nerves separate into smaller branches and enter the cord over much of the length of their spinal segment. The hallmark of spinal cord injury is the loss of movement and sensation below the level of the injury. This loss is typically partial at the level of injury because of three factors:

- The locations of the nerve cells involved in mediating sensation over any part of the body.
- The nerve cells that activate any muscle in the body are spread for a short distance along one or more spinal cord segments.
- At any spinal cord level, some sensory and motor functions that map to that level will be represented above the injury and some below.

Below the level of injury, the loss of function might be complete or partial, and the degree of functional loss is important in predicting the likelihood of recovery.

> The hallmark of spinal cord injury is the loss of movement and sensation below the level of the injury.

All of the parts of the nervous system have a degree of intrinsic ability to recover from injury, and this is true also of the spinal cord. In order to measure possible recovery, it is first necessary for the initial level and severity of injury to be determined. A neurologic examination is performed to assess sensation in different parts of the body and the strength of key muscles. The American Spinal Injury Association (ASIA) has adopted a widely accepted scoring system for this neurologic examination (Figure 1-7). The strength of each muscle is graded from 0 to 5, with 0 being totally paralyzed and 5 being normal. Sensation in the skin (*dermatomes*) represented by each spinal cord level is rated 0 if absent; 1 if impaired; and 2 if normal. The scores are added to give an overall motor and sensory score, which can indicate how much overall function has been preserved.

At any spinal cord level, the impact of an injury is determined by the degree of injury. A complete injury means that the patient has no preserved neurologic function below the level of injury. An incomplete injury means that some function is preserved below that level. A number

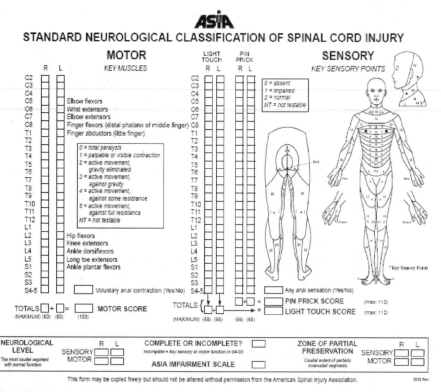

FIGURE 1-7

The Standard Neurologic Evaluation of the Spinal Cord Injured Patient.
Reproduced with permission of the American Spinal Injury Association.

Table 1-2 ASIA Adaptation of Frankel Classification

Class	Degree
A	**Complete.** All motor and sensory function is absent below the zone of partial preservation.
B	**Incomplete, preserved sensation only.** Preservation of any demonstrable, reproducible sensation, excluding phantom sensations. Voluntary motor functions are absent.
C	**Incomplete, preserved motor nonfunctional.** Preservation of voluntary motor function, which is minimal and performs no useful purpose. Minimal is defined as preserved voluntary motor ability below the level of injury, where the majority of the key muscles test at least a grade of 3 (for example, the muscle can move the limb sufficiently to oppose gravity).
D	**Incomplete, preserved motor functional.** Preservation of functionally useful voluntary motor function. This is defined as preserved voluntary motor ability below the level of injury, when the majority of the key muscles test at least a grade of 3.
E	**Complete return of all motor and sensory function.** At this level, a person might still have abnormal reflexes.

of rating scales have been devised to classify patients according to the completeness of a spinal cord injury. This permits doctors to monitor the progress of patients and predict the likelihood of significant recovery. The most widely accepted instrument for assessing the severity of SCI is the ASIA scale, an adaptation of the older Frankel Classifications (Table 1-2).

PROGNOSIS FOR SPINAL CORD INJURY

Immediately after SCI, there is a period of profound dysfunction due to a poorly understood phenomenon called *spinal shock*. During this period, all spinal cord reflexes, including the muscle stretch reflexes (Figure 1-4), are suppressed, whereas they will eventually be exaggerated, and the muscles are flaccid, whereas later they will be stiff. Spinal shock lasts from a few days to several weeks, and tends to last longer the more severe the injury. It appears that the recuperative ability of the nervous system relies on there being enough preserved structure to allow functional accommodation. Unless the initial impairment is so mild that improvement is not needed, the probability of functional recovery is greater the less complete the injury (Table 1-3).

According to reviews of the literature carried out by the Consortium for Spinal Cord Medicine, the chances that a person with an initial ASIA A classification will eventually regain the ability to walk, even with an assistive device such as a cane or walker, is only 3 percent.

> Immediately after SCI, there is a period of profound dysfunction due to a poorly understood phenomenon called *spinal shock*.

If sensation is preserved, including the ability to detect the sharpness of a pin in the area around the anus, the chances go up to 50 percent.

If the patient has some movement below the level of injury, even though the muscles are so weak that they cannot do anything useful, the chances of regaining the ability to walk go up to 75 percent. Additionally, if the muscles are strong enough to do useful things, such as raise the leg off the bed, the probability that the patient will eventually be able to walk is 95 percent.

Table 1-3 Correlation Between Initial ASIA Score and Probability of Functional Recovery

ASIA Score	Probability That a Person Will Regain the Ability to Walk With or Without an Assistive Device
A (Complete loss of motor and sensory function below the level of injury)	3 percent
B (Incomplete, preserved sensation only) with intact peri-anal pin sensation	50 percent
C (Incomplete, preserved nonfunctional motor)	75 percent
D (Incomplete, preserved functional motor)	95 percent

From: Consortium for Spinal Cord Medicine. *Outcomes following traumatic spinal cord injury: Clinical Practices Guidelines for Health-care Professionals.* Washington, DC: Paralyzed Veterans of America, 1999.

Obviously, the higher the level of injury, the larger the number of muscles that will be affected and the more area of skin that will lose sensation. Thus, the impact of SCI also depends on the level of the injury; this is reflected in the additional financial cost of living (see Table 2-1).

CHAPTER 2

Causes of Spinal Cord Injury and Dysfunction

S PINAL CORD INJURIES ARISE from many causes, both traumatic and disease-related. They can affect nearly two dozen different levels of the cord, and can produce modest to complete loss of movement and sensation below the level of injury. Thus, the outcomes and needs of those who suffer SCI differ from person to person. The two most common causes are trauma and ischemia.

TRAUMA

The average age for traumatic SCI is 29, with the most likely victim a male aged 18. Motor vehicle accidents account for nearly half of all cases. Acts of violence, such as gunshot wounds and stabbings, have risen as a cause in the U.S. in the past 25 years. More than 90 percent of sports-related injuries to the spinal cord from diving, football, gymnastics, and surfing cause *quadriplegia* (paralysis), because these types of injuries most often affect the cervical spine, and often penetrate the spinal cord.

When the injury is partial, the nature of the neurologic difficulties depends on what part of the spinal cord is severed. Figure 2-1B illus-

> The average age for traumatic SCI is 29, with the most likely victim a male aged 18.

trates a pure cut through the left side of the spinal cord (using X-ray images in which the anatomic part is assumed to be facing you). Of

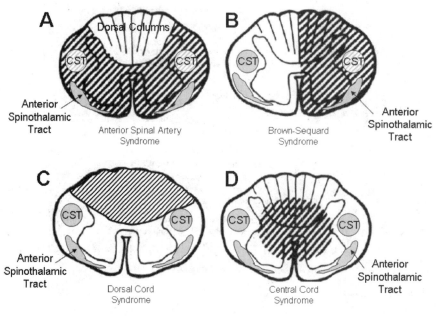

FIGURE 2-1

Incomplete Spinal Cord Syndromes. The nature of the neurologic deficits seen in partial spinal cord injuries depends on the type of injury and its location in the cross-section of the spinal cord. **A**, the anterior spinal artery syndrome is a "stroke" of the anterior (toward the front of the body; in the case of the spinal cord, also called "ventral") two thirds of the spinal cord, resulting from interruption of the blood supply through the anterior spinal artery. Note: Because the posterior (dorsal) part of the cord has many interdigitating arteries supplying it, a stroke of the dorsal cord is rare. **B**, the Brown-Sequard Syndrome is an injury to only one side of the spinal cord. It is named after a neurologist who described it in experimental animals. Such pure one-sided injuries are rare in real life, but approximate variations can be seen with knife wounds and other penetrating injuries and some tumors, such as certain benign tumors of the nerve roots. **C**, the dorsal cord syndrome is an injury most often resulting from compression of the cord by a metastatic tumor (a tumor originating from another part of the body that has invaded the blood stream and traveled to the cord) lodged in the rich network of veins on the dorsal (posterior, toward the back) surface of the spinal cord. **D**, the central cord syndrome is caused by non-penetrating injuries to the spine resulting in a "concussive" injury of the spinal cord. There is hemorrhage and cell death that begins in the center of the cord and spreads outward over several hours. A common cause is a whiplash injury, especially in older people whose spinal canals are narrowed by arthritis. Modified from: Cardenas DD and Warms C. Rehabilitation in Spinal Cord Injury. In: Selzer ME, Cohen LG, Gage FH, Clarke S, Duncan PW, eds, *Textbook of Neural Repair and Rehabilitation*, Cambridge University Press, 2006. After: Britell CW and Hammond MC. Spinal Cord injury. In: Hays RM, Kraft GH, Stolov WC, eds, *Chronic Disease Disability*, Demos Medical Publishing, 1994. **CST**=corticospinal tract.

course, such a precise *hemisection* of the spinal cord is rare in humans, but it can be produced in experimental animals. This is called the Brown-Séquard Syndrome, after the 19th century physiologist *Charles Edouard Brown-Séquard*, who first described it. The patient with a pure injury of this type would experience weakness and incoordination in the left side of the body below the injury because of the interruption of the corticospinal tract on the injured side. The ability to tell when an object is vibrating, or the position of a limb in space, is also lost on the left side because of the severance of the left dorsal columns.

By contrast, the ability to perceive pain or temperature would be lost on the right side below the injury, due to the interruption of the antero-lateral column, whose fibers have already crossed over from the opposite side of the spinal cord, as illustrated in Figure 1-5. Brown-Sequard syndrome might typically be caused by a knife or a bullet wound in which the point of entry was off center. Benign tumors of the coverings of the spinal cord or the nerve roots can compress the spinal cord from the side, also causing Brown-Séquard Syndrome.

Falls are another leading cause of SCI, especially in people over age 60. People with spinal canals narrowed by arthritis of the spine and disk disease or tumors can gradually worsen over months or years from compression of the cord. This often occurs at the neck or against the nerves that go to the legs and bladder, just beyond the lower tip of the spinal cord in the low back. The incidence ranges from 30–50 per million people around the world, with males outnumbering females 4:1, and the average age being 35 years old. The causes vary from country to country. Falls off a bicycle or cart in some regions will be more common than surfing and rock climbing accidents in others (Table 2-1).

In the cases of falls and motor vehicle accidents, the injury is most often caused by a hard blow (concussion) rather than penetration. The spinal cord is not pierced or torn by bone fragments, or an external projectile such as a bullet, but instead it is suddenly slammed against the inner surface of the boney spinal canal. At first, there might be no obvious abnormality in the spinal cord. However, during the hours after an injury, the central part of the spinal cord begins to hemorrhage and suffer destruction of nerve tissue, which spread outward over a period of about

Table 2-1 Incidence and Yearly Costs of SCI

Severity of Injury	Incidence	Yearly Added Health/Living Expense (estimated for 2005)
Quadriplegia		
Complete	19 percent	
C-1 to C-4		$115,000
C-5 to C-8		$47,000
Incomplete	30 percent	$14,000
Paraplegia		
Complete	28 percent	$24,000
Incomplete	21 percent	$13,000

This table indicates the proportion of spinal cord injuries that occur at different levels and whether they are complete or incomplete. Injuries are fairly uniformly distributed, although incomplete cervical injuries are most common. The higher the injury and the more complete, the greater the financial costs to patient and family. www.spinalcord.uab.edu.

2 days. The more severe the injury, the further outward the ultimate damage spreads. This gives rise to *central cord syndrome* (Figure 2-1D), which is described below in the section on *chronic cervical myelopathy*.

ISCHEMIA

As discussed in Chapter 1, ischemia (loss of blood flow) can affect the spinal cord. Sudden loss of blood flow to the spinal cord can occur during abdominal aortic surgery. A stroke can result from low blood flow or embolic debris that travels to the tiny arteries of the spinal cord, especially the thoracic cord. *Atherosclerosis* can narrow the inside of these arteries and cause a stroke of the spinal cord that can be sudden or progress over days.

The main artery that runs along the ventral (front) side of the spinal cord is called the *anterior spinal artery*. It supplies blood to the front two-thirds of the spinal cord (Figure 2-1A). A blockage of this artery produces weakness and loss of pain and temperature sensations below the level of the blockage, as predicted by the anatomic arrangement shown in Figure 1-6. The dorsal (back) part of the spinal cord receives blood through a highly branched network of arteries. No single artery blockage deprives the dorsal part of the spinal cord of blood. However, malignant tumors that spread via the bloodstream from other parts of the body (metasta-size), such as the lungs, breast, or prostate gland, often lodge in the veins located in front of the spinal cord, compressing the dorsal surface of the cord and producing loss of fine discrimination, vibration, and joint posi-tion sensations below the level of injury (Figure 2-1C).

Tumor growth further compresses the corticospinal tracts, causing weakness and incoordination below the injury. *Arteriovenous malforma-tions* (AVMs) of the cord are abnormal tangles of small arteries connect-ed directly to veins, in which the flow of blood is not slowed by the cap-illaries between them. These malformations gradually engorge with blood as the veins stretch. They can cause ischemia by taking blood away from the spinal cord tissue. They can also burst (hemorrhage)

> Many other neurologic diseases can cause symptoms of spinal cord dysfunction, and therefore present similar challenges with regard to long-term management and rehabilitation.

because the walls of veins are not thick enough to withstand the high pressure of arterial blood. They can cause single or recurrent bouts of loss of feeling or movement, usually in the legs.

Many other neurologic diseases can cause symptoms of spinal cord dysfunction, and therefore present similar challenges with regard to long-term management and rehabilitation.

CHRONIC CERVICAL MYELOPATHY

As we age, the spine becomes subject to the same types of arthritis as other joints. Wear and tear cause inflammation of the joints between adjacent spinal vertebrae, leading to buildup of calcium deposits and bony protrusions that can cause narrowing of the passageways by which the spinal nerves leave the spine (*spinal foramina*). This can give rise to pains radiating from the neck into the arms. The boney enlarge-ments also can cause narrowing of the spinal canal and squeezing of the spinal cord. Chronic compression of the spinal cord can cause neurolog-ical dysfunction, a disorder called *chronic cervical myelopathy*.

Most of the time, this type of deformity of the spinal cord occurs very slowly, and a person is able to adapt to it. The deep tendon reflexes might be brisk and the patient might experience some difficulty in walking or mild deterioration in coordination. However, because the spinal cord has no extra room to move, sudden neck flexion or extension, such as dur-ing a fall, can lead to bruising of the spinal cord and the development of central cord syndrome.

For reasons not completely understood, blunt trauma in which there is an impact to the spine without penetration of the spinal cord can cause a bruise to develop in the center of the spinal cord, leading to delayed swelling, bleeding, and nerve cell death. With time, this swelling spreads outward, causing death of the motor neurons in the injured segment, beginning with the neurons that control the upper arms and shoulders rather than those that control the hand. Interruption of motor and sensory fibers begin at the same level and work downward because the nerve fibers that represent the lower parts of the body are located outermost (Fig. 1-6). If the process stops before the injury is complete, the arms would be weakest and the legs might be spared.

This gives rise to the peculiar distribution of neurologic deficits known colloquially as the "man in a bottle" syndrome, because the shoulders might be profoundly weak and the patient might not be able to lift his arms up from his sides. However, in general, SCI can give rise to the same symptoms as acute spinal cord trauma, including weakness and numbness of the legs, stiffness and painful spasms of the legs, loss of bowel and bladder control, and unstable blood pressure.

From the time a person first sees a doctor for symptoms of cervical spondylosis, there are three equally possible outcomes:

- One-third will improve without assistance because the nervous sys-tem has intrinsic flexibility and can accommodate to anatomic injury.

- One-third will stay the same because the rate of anatomic deterioration will slow or stop to the point that physiologic adaptation mechanisms counterbalance the rate of anatomic deterioration.
- One-third will continue to get worse.

Neurologists are reluctant to recommend surgical remedies unless the patient has actual loss of strength or numbness at the level of the spondylosis or below it. Surgical approaches include:

- **Laminectomy**—chipping away the roof of the spinal canal to give the spinal cord more room
- **Percutaneous discectomy**—sucking out the jelly-like substance from the center of a herniated or severely bulging intervertebral disc
- **Foraminotomy**—chipping away the calcium deposits that are narrowing the intervertebral foramina and causing spinal nerve compression.

The details of these types of surgery are beyond the scope of this book, but they are less likely to be successful in relieving pain if there is no loss of power or sensation, and no electrical evidence for loss of muscle innervation on *electromyography*. This test involves inserting a needle electrode into the muscle while the patient contracts the muscle slightly, and recording the patterns of electricity generated by the muscle. This is probably because spondylotic changes are common as aging progresses, and most people do not experience symptoms. On the other hand, neck pain is very common, even in the absence of spondylosis. Therefore, when pain is the only symptom, there is less assurance that the structural abnormalities seen on X-rays or other imaging studies are the real cause; whereas, the patient might be risking surgical complications, such as infections, scar formation with worsening nerve damage, and rarely death resulting from complications of anesthesia.

LUMBAR SPINAL STENOSIS

The same arthritic changes that affect the cervical spine can affect the lumbar and sacral vertebrae. Thus, impingement of the spinal foramina pinches lumbar and sacral nerve roots, giving rise to shooting pains down the legs. Narrowing of the lumbar and sacral spinal canal does not cause spinal cord compression, because the spinal cord ends at the first lumbar vertebra. However, the spinal nerves of the cauda equina can be compressed, producing symptoms of cramping pain and weakness that come on or worsen with exercise, because the increased nerve activity elicits an increase in blood flow to the cauda equina and engorgement of veins that increases the pressure on the nerve roots. Laminectomy is the standard treatment.

TRANSVERSE MYELITIS

The spinal cord can be affected by inflammation, an immune system reaction that causes white blood cells and fluid to enter tissue from the blood because a foreign substance such as a virus or bacterium has been detected. Some white blood cells make antibodies and others ingest foreign substances. In most cases, no virus or other true foreign substance can be identified, and it is assumed that the immune system is reacting to the spinal cord itself. In particular, the immunologic attack seems to be directed against the myelin in what is assumed to be an autoimmune reaction. In other words, the immune system mistakes the myelin for a foreign substance.

> The spinal cord can be affected by inflammation, an immune system reaction that causes white blood cells and fluid to enter tissue from the blood because a foreign substance such as a virus or bacterium has been detected.

The reason for this is not known for certain. However, the swelling and other chemical reactions associated with inflammation can cause the spinal cord axons to lose their ability to conduct electrical impulses temporarily and mimic SCI. The symptoms build up over 1–2 days, and gradually decrease over several weeks as the swelling subsides. Afterwards, many of the affected axons can be interrupted, and some might have lost their myelin. Therefore, they will have an impaired ability to conduct electrical impulses. This gives rise to permanent partial spinal cord syndromes as in SCI.

Treatment generally consists of supportive care and intravenous administration of steroids such as methylprednisolone to reduce inflammation and hasten recovery. Most of the time, transverse myelitis is a solitary event that never recurs. However, in about one-third of cases (50 percent in women; 15 percent in men), people go on to have other episodes of neurologic inflammation in the spinal cord, brain, or optic nerves. These patients have multiple sclerosis.

MULTIPLE SCLEROSIS (MS)

MS is an immunological attack on myelin in the central nervous system—but not of the peripheral nerves. In 80 percent of cases, it consists of temporary attacks (remitting-exacerbating MS) in which neurologic dysfunction builds up rapidly over a few hours or days (exacerbations), and then there is partial improvement (remissions) over the next 2–4 weeks. Women are affected about twice as often as men, and the first attack usually occurs in the 20s or 30s. It is rare for a first attack to occur before adolescence or after the age of 50. About one-third of first attacks involve the spinal cord; one-third involve the optic nerves; and one-third involve the white matter of the brain, including the *cerebellum*.

The initial symptoms depend on which nerve fibers are involved. Attacks in the spinal cord can include numbness and weakness below the level of inflammation, inability to urinate, constipation, and sexual dysfunction. With each attack, a small amount of permanent damage remains after the inflammation and swelling have resolved. The accumulation of these residual deficits is what leads to long-term disability. As patients age, remissions tend to become less apparent, and the course of the disease tends to become chronically progressive (secondary-progressive MS).

Steroids such as prednisone and methylprednisolone can hasten remission, but there is little evidence that this reduces long-term cumulative disability. The number of attacks can be greatly reduced by preventative administration of *immunomodulatory* drugs, such as beta interferon, glatiramer acetate, mitoxantrone, and natalizumab. These medications are injected into the skin, muscle, or veins at different intervals from daily to every 3 months, depending on the drug. Evidence is accumulating that these treatments slow the long-term accumulation of disabilities. About 20 percent of cases never have a remitting and exacerbating course, but are chronically progressive from the beginning (primary-progressive MS). The effectiveness of immunomodulatory therapies in these cases is less well established.

OTHER CAUSES

Other diseases that can cause spinal cord dysfunction include:

- Amyotrophic lateral sclerosis (ALS, or Lou Gehrig's disease)
- Degeneration of the motor neurons in the spinal cord and their command neurons in the brain
- *Syringomyelia*, which is the development of a fluid-filled cavity in the center of the spinal cord (sometimes this develops at the site of a spinal cord injury and accounts for delayed worsening after the patient has recovered)
- Hereditary *spinocerebellar* degenerative diseases
- Syphilis of the spinal cord
- Vitamin B$_{12}$ deficiency
- Spinal cord abscesses caused by bacterial infections
- Spinal cord tumors

CHAPTER 3

Acute Treatment of Spinal Cord Injury

THE FIRST DAYS AFTER A TRAUMATIC SCI are devoted to protecting the injured tissue of the cord and the bodily functions of the injured person. Medical care that emphasizes prevention of complications and rapid treatment of problems that arise becomes a life-long pursuit for people who continue to have paralysis.

Remarkable improvements in life expectancy and in the ability to carry on a productive life have evolved, resulting in better training and

> The first days after a traumatic SCI are devoted to protecting the injured tissue of the cord and the bodily functions of the injured person.

care, treatments for infections and other medical conditions, rehabilitation, and assistive devices. For example, a quadriplegic person with a C6 level injury would have survived, on average, only 30 percent of the expected numbers of years in 1960, but due to advances in medical care and support systems, the survival rate was 60 percent of normal in 1980, and 81 percent in 2004. A person under the age of 30 who suffers SCI today has an even higher likelihood of a normal life expectancy.

Immediate Treatment by Emergency Medical Technicans

When a person has been injured and appears paralyzed, the police or other rescue workers are trained to suspect a spinal cord injury, and emergency medical technicians are dispatched to the scene. Their first efforts are aimed at keeping the injured person immobilized by placing them on a stable transporting board in a straight posture, supporting the head with sandbags or a similar device to make sure the neck does not bend or rotate, and making sure that the person can breathe. These personnel are usually trained to insert an airway, if necessary, and establish an intravenous route for the administration of medications. The patient is then transported to the hospital and, if possible, to one that is designated as a "level-1 trauma center" with staff experienced in SCI.

Initial Hospitalization

Radiologic Evaluation

Once the trauma patient is in the hospital, doctors and nurses will determine the type and severity of injuries. They will manage any medical problem that can compromise normal breathing and blood pressure, or produce further injury to the brain, spinal cord, and other organs. The spine is kept straight to prevent additional compression of the cord. If paralysis of the arms or legs is apparent from the initial examination, the location and extent of injury are assessed immediately by imaging.

Computerized tomography (CAT scan) and ordinary X-rays can show bone fractures and movement of bony elements surrounding the spinal cord that might have entered into the spinal canal. These tests do not show the substance of the spinal cord well, and might not reveal disk material that has slipped from between the vertebral bodies and is pressing against the cord.

Magnetic resonance imaging (MRI) reveals trauma outside and within the cord. Clotted blood, such as an *epidural hematoma* and fractured bones, are visible if they press against the cord. Edema or fluid that has swollen the cord, or a bloody hematoma leaking within the cord, can increase over several days. As previously discussed, these changes reflect an ongoing process of inflammation and biological response to impaired blood flow. Medical imaging cannot yet determine whether any of the ascending or descending axons have been spared within the region of swelling.

Persistently complete SCI occurs most often when:

- A hematoma is found within the substance of the cord
- There is displacement of the vertebral body so that it is wedged against the cord, especially at the T12–L1 level
- The joints (*facets*) of the cervical spine are detached or dislocated on their left and right sides
- A bullet is lodged within the canal.

Recovery is most common when the volume of injured spinal cord is small.

Treatment with Methylprednisolone

Clinical trials have suggested that intravenous injection of methylprednisolone within the first 8 hours of cord injury can modestly lessen the loss of movement and sensation, although the drug can cause side-effects. Use of this medication is still controversial, in part because the clinical trials performed to establish its effectiveness included a relatively small number of subjects who had a wide range of injuries and did not differ in their functional outcomes. Therefore, it was not clear whether the clinical trials could adequately discriminate between the effectiveness of the medication compared to a placebo. Nevertheless, the administration of a large dose of methylprednisolone intravenously during the first 8 hours, and then in a slow drip for the next 24 hours has become standard practice in most hospitals.

Surgical Decompression and Stabilization

From 50–70 percent of patients in North America have spinal surgery after SCI. The timing might depend upon other medical complications, but the tendency in North America is to operate within the first 24–72 hours to reduce pressure on the spinal cord and remove bone fragments. Aligning the bones of the spinal column is a long-term goal (Figure 3-1), in order to prevent future mechanical deformities such as *scoliosis* and, in the case of a lumbar injury, to enhance the stability of the patient's cen-

> The specific type of surgical approach depends upon the level and extent of injury, and the experience of the surgeon.

ter of gravity in order to facilitate walking. Surgeons also hope to prevent future injuries of the spinal cord and eliminate potential spinal sources of pain.

The specific type of surgical approach depends upon the level and extent of injury, and the experience of the surgeon. Research is needed to better define the need for surgery, because all surgery carries risks, even if there is no neurologic function to lose because the SCI is already complete. For example, the postoperative wound can become infected, as indicated by reddened areas around the sutures and leakage of fluid.

Non-Surgical Immobilization

In some countries, traction and other immobilization techniques are more widely used than surgical stabilization. Until recently, it has not been clear that surgery is preferable to more conservative methods for most patients. However, very recent evidence suggests an advantage to the earliest possible decompression of the spinal cord and stabilization of the spinal column. Stiff collars that prevent more than a few degrees of neck motion after cervical injures often suffice, but some patients might need to wear a rigid external halo brace attached to the skull and to a molded vest to allow for healing of bone grafts.

A custom-molded, thermoplastic body jacket might be needed after a *thoracolumbar* injury to limit spine mobility. Collars, vests, and casted limbs can compromise early rehabilitation efforts for mobility and self-

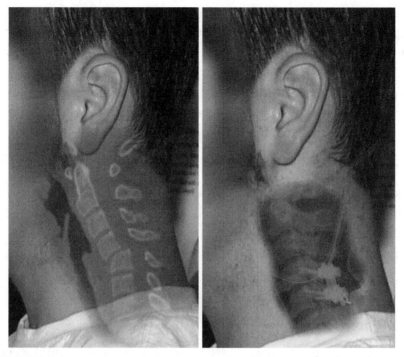

FIGURE 1-3

Surgical alignment of injured cervical spine after SCI. This patient has had an injury that caused dislocation of the spine. In these pictures, the X-ray images are superimposed on the photographs. Notice in the left- hand frame how the 5th and 6th vertebrae are not aligned smoothly. This is corrected surgically in the right-hand frame, in which the surgical hardware is also visible.

care tasks because they restrict head and trunk movements. These devices also predispose the patient to pressure sores and shallow breathing with pneumonia, so preventative efforts are needed. Surgeons usually remove these stabilizers by 4–12 weeks after SCI, making transfers and lower body care easier.

Prevention of Blood Clots in Veins

Small blood clots tend to form in the veins of the legs and pelvis when normal mobility is interrupted. Paralysis and bed rest can lead to clots, which are called *deep vein thromboses* (DVTs). These clots cause the leg to swell with fluid and become tender. If the clots break free and travel to the lungs (*pulmonary embolism*), they can prevent the lungs from absorbing oxygen from the air, leading to heart and lung damage, and even death.

The risk for these complications can be reduced by placing the legs inside plastic sleeves into which air is pumped intermittently, producing intermittent pneumatic leg compression. This causes the blood in the leg veins to keep moving and return to the heart. DVTs are also prevented by twice a day administration of an injected anticoagulant such as heparin or enoxaparin. These interventions will continue until the patient is able to stand and walk—about 2–3 months, which is usually through the end of inpatient rehabilitation. If trauma to the legs or pelvis has occurred, or if venous thrombosis or pulmonary emboli are detected by tests despite preventative measures, a higher dose of an anticoagulant is given for 6 or more months.

Respiration

Breathing requires coordinated movements of the muscles of the chest, abdomen, and diaphragm in order to contract and expand the lungs. Carbon dioxide is breathed out as the muscles relax and the lungs contract. A voluntary or reflexive cough requires forceful exhalation to clear the airways of mucous, help prevent pneumonia, and make eating and drinking safer.

The ability to carry out ordinary breathing and coughing requires proper functioning of the nerves and muscles from C4 to T10. Lesions (anatomical abnormalities due to injury or disease) at or above C4 affect the diaphragm, the neck muscles, and all the muscles at lower spinal levels. C5 to C8 lesions, and to a lesser extent T1 to T10 injuries, affect the intercostal muscles (muscles between the ribs that assist inspiration by elevating the rib cage), and some of the shoulder and abdominal muscles that normally expand the chest and lungs. The diaphragm, however, works well enough to maintain at least daytime ventilation unless fatigue develops.

The main dangers resulting from impaired action and coordination of these muscles include inadequate oxygen getting to the brain and other organs, and the development of pneumonia. Lung infections often occur soon after SCI as a result of collapse of some of the tiny air pock-

> The ability to carry out ordinary breathing and coughing requires proper functioning of the nerves and muscles from C4 to T10.

ets within the lungs (*alveoli*), and because of breathing secretions and bacteria from the mouth and upper airways down into the lungs, a dysfunction called *aspiration*. Indeed, pneumonia is one of the greatest threats to quadriplegic patients (resulting from cervical SCI) throughout life, and a persistent if lesser threat to those with paraplegia from a thoracic SCI. At least 20 percent of deaths in the months and years after SCI are due to pulmonary infections. They are most common in people with higher complete lesions and in people over 60 years old.

If a *tracheostomy* was necessary to best manage ventilation soon after SCI, people with an injury below C4 are likely to gradually be weaned successfully from the tracheostomy tube and ventilator once they learn to cough well enough to clear lung secretions and contract their breathing muscles. Sometimes, the initial trauma and cervical surgery cause swelling of tissues and the vocal cords (*glottis*). This swelling must diminish before the ability to manage secretions and swallowing can improve. Light chest percussion (tapping) over the ribcage and postural drainage by lowering the patient's head can loosen and move secretions that can plug the small airways and lead to infections behind the plugged passage or collapsed lung spaces. Suctioning mucous from a tracheostomy or the back of the throat can induce an exaggerated reflex in the *vagus nerve* (the nerve that runs from the brainstem down the neck and chest to supply motor and sensory function to several vital organs, including the heart), resulting in dangerous, extreme slowing of the heart, so caution is necessary, especially in the first month after SCI. Sometimes a medication such as atropine is needed to counteract slowing of the heart by blocking the action of the neurotransmitter acetylcholine on the heart.

Doctors can assess breathing function by measuring the maximum pressures generated in the airway during inspiration and expiration, along with the maximum volume of air that the patient can inhale and exhale (the vital capacity and forced expiratory volume). The levels of oxygen in the blood are measured by *finger oximetry*, using a clip-on device that translates the redness of the blood in the finger into oxygen concentration, and by blood tests.

These bedside tests tend to correlate with the voluntary ability to cough and breathe efficiently. If normal breathing is insufficient, intermittent positive pressure breathing (IPPB) through the tracheostomy will be necessary. Long-term, this mechanical approach is effective, but many complications can arise, and suctioning of secretions is often required.

Exercise such as inspiratory resistive training, sometimes performed with some type of feedback, can strengthen the breathing muscles—the diaphragm, *trapezius, sternocleidomastoid* and chest wall muscles—that are still functioning. Postural support from the nerves and muscles of the diaphragm, neck, and trunk also must be improved. Some quadriplegic patients benefit from the daily practice of doing forced inspiration and expiration exercises. Muscles that are ordinarily not very involved in breathing and coughing can be brought into a more supportive role. For example, the upper *pectoral* and abdominal muscles can be trained for expiration during a cough. Training must take into account movements of the chest wall that can hinder breathing.

Pressure and support of the abdomen by a binder can place the diaphragm into a better position when the patient is seated and increase lung volume. Intermittent pressure over the abdomen can improve the force of a cough, but it should not be used when the patient is lying on her back. The rib cage can stiffen over time if increased muscle tone and too little physical activity decrease its flexibility. This can lessen the contributions of the chest wall muscles to breathing. Some people, particularly former smokers, benefit from medications that cause relaxation of the smooth muscles of the airways because they elicit bronchodilation. For people who can be maintained off of a ventilator during the day, or who develop *sleep apnea* during the night, *biphasic positive airway pressure*

(BIPAP) can be provided by a nasal mask to support inspiratory and expiratory pressures. Some high quadriplegic people can be helped by other devices, such as a corset that inflates cyclically (a *pneumo-belt*) when they are seated, and an electrical stimulator that is applied to the *phrenic nerve* of the diaphragm. Considerable monitoring must accompany these approaches.

CHAPTER 4

Health Care After SCI

S PINAL CORD INJURIES are disabling because mobility is lost, but other impairments of SCI are equally troublesome and can be more dangerous to health and survival. These impairments involve faulty regulation of vital functions we are not usually aware of because they are automatic and do not require conscious behavior on our part. The autonomic nervous system that controls blood pressure, heart rate, temperature, and other involuntary vital functions. The autonomic nervous system includes:

1. **The sympathetic nervous system**, which exits the central nervous system in the thoracic and lumbar ventral roots and uses norepinephrine as its neurotransmitter. Norepinephrine *speeds* the heart rate and increases the force of heart contraction, raising blood pressure.
2. **The parasympathetic nervous system**, which exits the central nervous system at the level of the brainstem and sacral spinal cord, and uses acetylcholine as its neurotransmitter. Acetylcholine slows the heart rate and lowers blood pressure.

Like the voluntary nervous system, the autonomic nervous system receives descending neural control from the brain. The loss of descending controls compromises these vital autonomic reflexes. Disturbance of the hormones released by glands that are ordinarily under autonomic nervous

> Spinal cord injuries are disabling because mobility is lost, but other impairments of SCI are equally troublesome and can be more dangerous to health and survival.

system control, and the release of norepinephrine, which ordinarily maintains the blood pressure and heart rate, also compromise the smooth regulation of body temperature and blood sugar. Early after SCI, the main problem is an insufficient amount of sympathetic nervous system activity.

BLOOD PRESSURE AND HEART RATE

With SCI above T6, there is a tendency for the blood pressure to decrease when a person sits with the legs over the side of a bed or chair, and when standing. The normal reflexes that maintain blood pressure when blood pools in the legs—and the heart has to pump blood against gravity—include a more efficient contraction of the heart muscle, constriction of the blood vessels, especially in the abdomen, and an increase in the heart rate. These are all disturbed with high SCI. This sudden decrease in blood pressure when sitting or standing (20 mm or more of mercury) is called *orthostatic hypotension* (OH), and it can result in dizziness, wooziness, a sense of imminent loss of consciousness, slowed thinking, fatigue, and fainting.

Low blood sugar and many other medical problems can cause the same symptoms, so the best way to check blood pressure and heart rate is while lying flat, and then after sitting with the legs dangling or after standing for several minutes. It is especially important to check these vital signs during the first sessions of sitting and standing, as well as during early rehabilitation therapies.

The following simple measures can help prevent or reduce the severity of OH:

- Take oral fluids and salt to increase blood volume.
- Use elastic leg wraps to prevent pooling of blood in veins.
- Practice moving upright gradually to help restore some of the normal reflexes.
- Lie on a bed angled 5 degrees or more so that the heels are lower than the head, which helps the kidneys retain fluid overnight.

Several medications help retain salt or constrict the blood vessels to stabilize the blood pressure. Some people will need to keep a digital blood pressure cuff at home to monitor their pressures and adjust the management. Blood pressure can rise too high during time spent in bed using methods that retain salt and water, so a short-acting, nighttime, antihypertensive medication might be necessary. Severe headaches are a symptom that this is happening.

OH can also be managed using these simple methods:

- Keep well hydrated during the day.
- Wrap legs moderately tightly with an elastic material, starting from the ball of the foot and working up to the knee.
- Sleep in the reverse Trendelenburg position (buttocks down, head up, knees slightly bent, feet slightly raised)—raise the head of the bed 4–6 inches by placing planks on the floor under the bed frame, or by tilting an electric hospital bed. Monitor for skin reddening.
- Add a salt tablet (1 gram of sodium) to each meal.
- Take Florinef® (fludrocortisone acetate); 0.1 mg in the morning to retain salt and water.
- Take midodrine; 5–10 mg when out of bed, every 4–6 hours as needed to increase blood pressure.

BODY TEMPERATURE

Body temperature is maintained, even in a cool environment, by the release of hormones, by shivering to make heat, and by constriction of the blood vessels (*vasoconstriction*) in the skin to limit heat loss. After SCI above T6, loss of muscle mass and autonomic reflexes for vasoconstriction can lead to low body temperatures (*hypothermia*) in cool environments and high body temperatures (*hyperthermia*) in warm environments. For cold feet, wool socks can be worn to help retain warmth.

BLADDER DYSFUNCTION

Immediately after SCI, the bladder cannot be emptied because the normal reflexes that cause the bladder to contract are suppressed. Urine is retained because the internal sphincter muscle located at the outflow of the bladder into the urethra, and the external sphincter muscle located around the urethra itself are in a constant state of contraction, which closes off the outflow pathway. As urine forms in the kidneys, it flows down to the bladder through collecting tubes called *ureters*.

Once the bladder fills with urine, it empties automatically because sensory nerve fibers in the bladder wall detect the expansion of the bladder and activate local spinal cord reflexes that cause the sphincter muscles to relax and the *detrusor* muscles in the bladder wall to contract (Figure 4-1). The nerves for the bladder and its sphincters are located at two spinal cord levels, T11-L1 and S2-S4. However, these spinal cord control centers are controlled by descending inputs from the brain, so after a spinal cord injury the ability to coordinate bladder activity is at least temporarily lost. The muscles of the bladder wall and the outlet sphincters might not sense the fullness of the bladder and not contract in order to express urine.

If emptying does not occur, the pressure in the bladder builds up and urine backs up into the ureters and kidneys. Pain, infection from stagnation of urine, and kidney failure can develop. Several methods are employed to prevent these complications. Intermittent catheterization is performed with either a clean reusable catheter or a sterile catheter, especially in a hospital setting. Patients learn how to insert the catheter into the urethra when the bladder fills beyond 300–400 cc. In the hospital, ultrasound testing can be used to detect fullness.

Great care must be taken to avoid introducing bacteria from the hands or skin near the urethral opening into which the catheter is inserted. Cleanliness helps prevent urinary tract infections. If an intermittent catheterization program (ICP) is uncomfortable or difficult for a person with quadriplegia to manage, an indwelling (*Foley*) catheter can be left in the bladder. A catheter can also be surgically placed above the boney pubis (the front part of the pelvic bone) through the lower abdomen (*suprapublic cystostomy*).

Cleanliness helps prevent urinary tract infections.

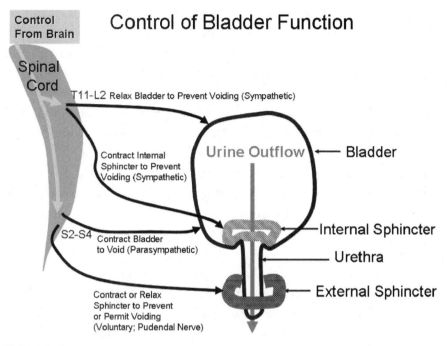

Control of Bladder Function

Control From Brain

Spinal Cord

T11-L2 Relax Bladder to Prevent Voiding (Sympathetic)

Contract Internal Sphincter to Prevent Voiding (Sympathetic)

Urine Outflow ←—— Bladder

S2-S4 Contract Bladder to Void (Parasympathetic)

Internal Sphincter

Urethra

Contract or Relax Sphincter to Prevent or Permit Voiding (Voluntary; Pudendal Nerve)

External Sphincter

FIGURE 4-1

The Lower Spinal Cord Controls the Bladder. Nerves arising at two spinal cord levels control urination. At T11-L2, nerves of the sympathetic nervous system have two effects that keep the urine in the bladder, thereby preventing incontinence. First, they cause relaxation of the detrusor muscle in the bladder wall, so that the bladder does not contract. Second, they cause the internal sphincter muscle to contract, preventing leakage of urine out of the bladder into the urethra. At the S2-S4 levels, nerves of the parasympathetic nervous system have the opposite effect. They trigger urination by causing contraction of the detrusor muscles in the bladder wall and simultaneously relaxing the internal sphincter muscle. A nerve of voluntary control, the *pudendal* nerve, also arises at the S2-S4 level and controls the muscles of the pelvic floor, including the external urethral sphincter. When this nerve is activated, these muscles contract and prevent urine from passing out through the urethra. Thus, voluntary relaxation of these muscles is necessary for normal urination. Sensory nerve fibers that travel from the bladder to the spinal cord through all these nerves provide information to the brain about the state of bladder filling, and also trigger reflex emptying when the bladder is full.

Over time, people whose SCI is above T12 can develop reflexive bladder. This means that when the bladder fills even a little, it suddenly contracts and empties, often without warning. This incontinence can be managed in men by using an external condom catheter.

For urination to be effective, the contraction of the detrusor muscle of the bladder wall must be coordinated with relaxation of the sphincters. These two components act synergistically. In people with SCI, this coordination can be lost or incomplete, and the sphincter muscles do not relax as the bladder wall contracts. This is called *detrusor-sphincter dyssynergia*, which means that urine cannot escape easily, and only small amounts of urine are released or leak. In people with a lesion of the *conus medullaris* below T12, the nerve cells from S2 to S4 can be lost and the bladder will lose the motor nerve cells that cause detrusor contraction and internal sphincter relaxation. The bladder will not contract at all, and will continue to fill until catheterized.

Storage problems

A leaky bladder can cause skin breakdown and social embarrassment. A relaxant medication such as oxybutynin can increase the capacity of the bladder and lessen the possibility of leaking. However, if the bladder wall cannot contract enough, this can lead to the need for catheterization. *Dyssynergia* can be managed with similar medication in combination with other medicines, such as terazosin to relax the internal sphincter in the neck of the bladder. A newer approach is to inject botulinum toxin into the bladder to lessen detrusor muscle overactivity. People who cannot store urine can improve their bladder functioning by performing pelvic muscle exercises, if possible. Enlargement of the bladder can be performed surgically. More often, patients with lesions above T12 can benefit from sacral nerve root stimulation using a device such as the Vocare™ after the sensory nerve roots are cut to interrupt reflex emptying. In one study of the Vocare™, the number of urinary tract infections, catheter use, reflex incontinence, the need for anticholinergic medication, and dysreflexia were all reduced, compared to intermittent catheterization. Of course, every surgical procedure has its potential complications. Placing a Vocare™ device can be complicated by bleeding, wound infections, mechanical problems due to formation of scar tissue, and other undesirable consequences.

Emptying problems

As indicated above, incomplete emptying can lead to increased backup pressure on the kidneys, which can cause kidney damage. Moreover, if the bladder does not empty completely, urine remains stagnant, which allows time for bacteria to grow and establish a bladder infection. As a general rule, in order to prevent backup pressure from causing kidney disease, the volume of urine in the bladder should not exceed 400 cc. In order to avoid infections, the amount of urine remaining in the bladder after voiding (the *residual volume*) should not exceed 100 cc.

Scheduled times are set to void and if this is not successful, intermittent catheterization is performed. The time schedule will be adjusted based on drinking habits. Usually four catheterizations per day are enough. If medications do not lead to adequate emptying in people with dyssynergia, the sphincter can be surgically cut to make it incompetent, or a mesh stent can be inserted into the urethra.

The same catheter can be reused if it is kept clean using a mild soap, rinsed, and dried in a plastic bag before sealing the bag. Boiling or microwaving a catheter is not necessary. A touch of lubricating gel can make insertion easier. Many brands of single-use catheters, some that

> Urological evaluation of the kidneys should be performed yearly for people using catheters, and more often if infections, kidney stones, or other complications recur.

are pre-lubricated, are available, and experimentation will lead to the most acceptable choice. It is important to drink at least 2 liters of fluid during the day. By not drinking after dinner, most people can sleep a full night after their final evening catheterization. At home, the adequacy of bladder emptying can be monitored in people who appear to be voiding spontaneously by checking a few residual volumes. This is done after voiding by inserting a catheter into the bladder through the urethra, collecting the urine in a measuring container, and measuring the volume.

Drinking cranberry juice or taking acidifying tablets can lessen the ability of bacteria to cling to the inner wall of the bladder and cut down on infections. Infections become easy to spot. A change in the smell or the clarity of the urine, bladder irritation that causes spontaneous leaking or muscle spasms, fever, and dysreflexia are warning signs.

Urological evaluation of the kidneys should be performed yearly for people using catheters, and more often if infections, kidney stones, or other complications recur.

BOWEL DYSFUNCTION

Food that is eaten passes down through the esophagus and then into the stomach and small intestine, where it is digested. The digested food is absorbed into the bloodstream, and the waste products of digestion remain in the alimentary canal, where they move through the large bowel and rectum, until finally being eliminated through the anus. Food and feces are moved along through this process by slow contractions called *peristalsis*. These contractions are induced by involuntary neural controls, with voluntary nerves to the anal sphincter contributing to control of defecation. Unlike the bladder, the alimentary canal has an intrinsic nervous system with a very complex pharmacology, which is capable of functioning on its own to move food and waste without any spinal cord input. This intrinsic nervous system contains about 100 million neurons, about as many as in the spinal cord. Nevertheless, the motility of the alimentary canal is strongly influenced by the autonomic nervous system, with some additional voluntary control.

The autonomic nervous system has more complex functions than can be summarized here, but in general, the sympathetic nervous system slows peristalsis, and the parasympathetic nervous system accelerates it. After SCI, constipation develops because the motility of the bowel slows as the result of an imbalance between sympathetic and parasympathetic activity. If constipation is severe, stool accumulating at the point of lost peristalsis becomes hard and totally blocks the bowel (stool impaction). In addition, voluntary contraction and relaxation of the sphincters can be lost, and incontinence of feces can occur.

Bowel programs should be adjusted based on diet and the consistency of the stool. In general, a program should include administration of stool softeners such as docusate twice a day, a motility enhancing agent such as senna, and a bisacodyl suppository at night to promote a morning bowel movement. An enema might be needed if no bowel movement has occurred for several days. Rectal stimulation with a gloved finger, or a glycerin suppository, can help initiate a morning bowel movement. If the SCI is below T12, manual removal of stool might be necessary because the rectum has lost its motility.

When stools are loose or incontinence is a problem, wearing a diaper, adding fiber to the diet, and reducing consumption of some of the foods that increase bowel motility (caffeine, berries, vitamins, high lactose loads, glutens, etc.) will help eliminate the problem. Occasional incontinence might seem like a social catastrophe, but friends and family will understand.

Like a bladder program, it takes time and some experimentation to develop a bowel program. Changes in diet and gas-forming foods can upset the regularity of bowel movements. Many medications, including the anticholinergics that lessen bladder contractions, antispasticity agents, narcotic pain medications, and some antidepressants, can depress bowel motility and cause constipation. Two quarts of fluid a day, fiber from foods or supplements, and exercise will help keep the stool soft.

If, in rare instances, repeated incontinence leads to soiling and pressure sores, or if a bowel program simply cannot be developed, a surgical colostomy can be performed. A pouch of colon is surgically brought to the abdomen and opens to a collection bag that is easily emptied.

INTELLECTUAL DYSFUNCTION

Up to half of the people who experience serious SCI will have had a traumatic or *hypoxic* (lack of oxygen) brain injury at the same time, or they might have impairment of memory, learning, concentration, and behavior from a prior brain injury. Repeated examinations of thinking processes and neuropsychological testing might be necessary to detect and manage these problems. Otherwise, these impairments can limit progress in self-care; for example, by the patient's forgetting to check their skin and take medications. This, in turn, can interfere with successful return to school or work.

DYSREFLEXIA OR DYSAUTONOMIA

Just as interruption of descending spinal cord pathways can lead to loss of inhibition of muscle reflexes and cause spasticity, interruption of descending control of autonomic reflexes can lead to loss of normal inhibition of autonomic reflexes, and to severe abnormalities of vital functions. This is called *autonomic dysreflexia*, or *dysautonomia*. In people with severe or complete lesions above the mid-thoracic cord, the normal inhibition of sympathetic outflow can be lost. This causes exaggeration of the reflexes that normally manage how much the blood vessels constrict in controlling blood pressure. Moreover, because the sympathetic innervation of the entire body, including the head, comes from the thoracic and lumbar spinal cord segments, abnormal sympathetic reflexes can even affect parts of the body above the level of injury.

Symptoms of episodic dysreflexia include pounding headache, fear and anxiety, sweating, flushing, and goose bumps above the injury level. In addition, dangerously slow heartbeat with marked rise in blood pressure can occur, which stresses the heart. The blood pressure can abruptly rise above 180/100, and the heart rate can simultaneously fall below 60.

Occasionally, autonomic dysreflexia occurs during the first several weeks after SCI. This is usually caused by fecal impaction, urine infection, a bladder or bowel distention, or an unrecognized bone fracture below the level of sensation in people with a high cervical injury. Bouts of dysreflexia are more common beginning about 3 months after SCI. Studies have related autonomic dysreflexia to any aggravation of chronic pain, bouts of more intense pain, muscle spasms, infections, full bladder, and constipation. Painful or irritating stimuli, such as those that can aggravate spasticity, must be identified and eliminated. This can be difficult because if the painful condition occurs at a level below the injury, the patient does not feel the pain, and therefore will be unable to locate the cause.

A distended rectum or bladder must be emptied. This is best accomplished with an anesthetic gel if digital stimulation is necessary to empty the bowels, or with a lubricated bladder catheter to lessen irritation. An antibiotic must be used if bladder infection is suspected. A distended, gaseous bowel can be managed by passing the gas, taking simethicone, and looking for dietary causes. Tight clothing such as a belt, bra, underwear, or shoes must be loosened. Pressure caused by the seat of the wheelchair must be relieved, and the legs must be uncrossed if dysreflexia occurs in bed. The patient should be examined for an ingrown toenail, skin injury or breakdown (even a sunburn or skin irritation from a hot water burn), or a tender or inflamed joint. Menstrual cramps and pregnancy, especially labor, as well as sexual arousal and orgasm also can cause dysreflexia.

If no cause is found, the doctor should look for a medical problem in the chest or abdomen, such as a mucus plug, stomach ulcer, or inflamed appendix. A new fracture of a bone in the foot or leg, and an unstable vertebral body from loosening of surgical hardware at the site of the injury, can be contributing factors. An enlarging fluid-filled space within the cord (*syrinx*) can also induce repeated bouts of dysautonomia that begin long after SCI.

The medications given for extreme *hypertension* (high blood pressure) must be managed cautiously to avoid causing a profound fall in the blood pressure and subsequent fainting. If the injured person is highly susceptible to dysreflexia, it is wise to keep a digital blood pressure cuff in the home to monitor pressure when using a new medication given by a doctor. If dysreflexia occurs while supine (lying on the back), the patient should sit up with their legs over the side of the bed or chair, in order to lessen the return of blood from the legs to the heart, which will lower the pressure. Useful drugs for people with recurrent bouts of hypertension greater than 200/110 include nitropaste, labetalol and nifedipine.

FATIGUE OR WEAKNESS

Weakness refers to the inability of a muscle or group of muscles to contract with normal force, resulting in the inability to carry out the normal tasks associated with those muscles. A muscle might be normal in strength when performing a one-time task, but lose strength with repeated action. This is called *muscle fatigue*. Even normal muscles can become fatigued if they are overused. Low levels of fitness make the activities of all muscles more difficult to maintain. In this sense, fatigue can apply not just to one set of muscles, but to the whole body.

> *Weakness* refers to the inability of a muscle or group of muscles to contract with normal force, resulting in the inability to carry out the normal tasks associated with those muscles.

Poor sleep, hot weather, medical complications such as anemia and heart and lung disease, certain medications, and depression can add to becoming easily fatigued during daily activity, especially as the day wears on. There are many forms of fatigue: the development of actual weakness in a muscle or muscles, physiological lack of stamina, and psychological lack of energy. People with SCI should try to describe their symptoms to the doctor so as to distinguish between weakness and fatigue, and between the various forms of fatigue. This can be done by describing symptoms within the context of how the day is spent, in other words, the functions of daily living associated with fatigue.

Causes of fatigue
After SCI, sleep apnea is remarkably frequent. Breathing is repeatedly interrupted, the brain is robbed of oxygen, and sleep is not refreshing. This leads to general fatigue during the day. Urinary urgency and pain also interrupt sleep. However, if shortness of breath with modest exertion accompanies fatigue, it can be a sign of a cardiac problem or a lung disorder. A physical exam and special tests to evaluate heart and lung function might be necessary. SCI patients should try to increase their exercise tolerance gradually by pushing their wheelchair, and by per-

forming arm and leg exercises, whenever possible, in order to build up an energy reserve.

Physical fitness and improved management of high blood pressure, diabetes, and abnormal cholesterol ratios can be achieved, in part, by exercise that gets the heart rate above 60 percent of the difference between 220 and the person's age for one-half hour, four times per week. For example, a 50-year-old SCI patient should exercise hard enough to get their heart rate above (220–50) × 0.6 = 102/min. for 30 minutes, four times per week. Some people with electrical conduction abnormalities and other heart problems might not be able to do this, and a medical evaluation should be performed to establish a safe exercise regimen.

Any decline in strength requires further evaluation. Many of the complications discussed in this chapter can further weaken muscle strength and functional use of the arms, trunk and legs. Some of the treatable causes are non-use of muscle groups because of joint pain, spasms, or dysreflexia; lack of an exercise regimen that aims to maintain or increase the reserves for activities; and syringomyelia. Endocrine (glandular and hormonal) problems such as thyroid disease can weaken muscle.

Medications can also impair strength. For example, elevated cholesterol levels can accompany inactivity with genetic predisposition. The cholesterol-lowering statin drugs and other medicines can cause muscle damage (*myopathy*), with muscle weakness that can add to disability. A pinched nerve at the wrist or elbow can cause pain and worsen hand weakness. Problems that are common in anyone with aging, such as a peripheral neuropathy from diabetes or compression of a nerve root (*radiculopathy*) from a herniated intervertebral disk, can complicate the effects of SCI.

Actual weakness must be separated from a sense of fatigue, and difficulty in home and community activities from malaise, poor sleep, and depression. A doctor who is accustomed to managing people with SCI and other neurologic diseases might be needed to sort out these difficulties.

MOOD DISORDERS

Anxiety and depression can develop at any time after SCI. These mood disorders are common in the general population, and in people with new disabilities of any type. Depression is no more frequent in people with SCI than in people with other medical problems. Stressors such as pain, reduced social activity, personal and family problems, and cognitive difficulties from head trauma at the time of injury can contribute to depression. People with a history of depression or of drug and alcohol abuse are more likely than the general population to experience increased depression after SCI.

The symptoms of depression include:

- Difficulty concentrating
- Poor sleep
- Recurrent negative thoughts
- Feeling blue
- Diminished energy and appetite
- Inability to find pleasure
- Thoughts of suicide

Symptoms of depression should be discussed openly with the doctor and family. Depression almost always responds to developing a stronger social support network, antidepressant medications, and talk therapy with a professional.

NUTRITIONAL DIFFICULTIES

Muscle breaks down during bed rest at the rate of about 1 percent per 1–2 days, until about 10–15 percent of the muscle mass is lost. During the first few weeks after SCI, the physiologic stress of fever, poor nutrition, diarrhea, and the other physical insults that commonly afflict people with SCI cause a general *catabolic state*—a condition in which protein and other large molecules are broken down and converted to energy. This adds to the loss of muscle, atrophy of immobile muscles, and weight loss. Blood tests for pre-albumin and albumin can help determine the state of nutritional proteins.

The integrity of the skin depends on optimal nutrition. Tube feedings from commercially prepared mixes can be used early after SCI when swallowing is impaired. They contain the vitamins and proteins needed

The integrity of the skin depends on optimal nutrition.

if enough liquid can be used without causing diarrhea or reflux of fluid from the stomach into the esophagus. The regular diet should include vegetables, fruits, and nuts for fiber content, and should be adjusted to prevent weight gain outside of the range of the person's ideal weight. Low levels of activity can predispose to diabetes, hypertension, and abnormal levels of cholesterol. These problems require close supervision by a doctor.

OSTEOPOROSIS

Hormonal changes and immobility cause an average loss of 33 percent of the calcium from the bones below the level of the injury by 6 months after SCI. The rapid entry of calcium into the bloodstream can result in abnormally high blood calcium levels during the first few weeks after SCI, requiring medical attention. Ultimately, however, the calcium is excreted in the urine. The loss of calcium predisposes the person with SCI to fractures of the long bones of the legs. Voluntary exercise of the leg muscles and walking can help prevent calcium loss. When complete paralysis is present, however, functional electrical stimulation of leg muscles against the resistance of bicycle pedals and weight-supported treadmill training can have a limited effect on restoring bone mass. Medication such as calcitriol, a form of vitamin D, might be required to prevent excessive calcium loss.

PAIN

Pain is one of the more disabling problems for many people after SCI, especially when it is chronic and occurs daily. Pain can interfere with daily activities, sleep, and the sense of well-being. It can arise from many different and interacting sources, which must be identified and treated.

HETEROTOPIC OSSIFICATION

Sometimes bone is deposited in the muscles and tendons—mostly in the region of the hip, shoulder, or scapula—after a period of swelling or inflammation. If not recognized, this *heterotopic ossification* (HO) can increase, causing pain, limiting the range of motion of the nearby joints, and limiting use of an arm or leg. HO starts soon after SCI, but might not be noticed because of other complications and the fact that the person cannot feel pain below the injury. Any area of the body that becomes tender, warm, and painful should be quickly treated for potential HO with anti-inflammatory drugs, such as ibuprofen, and range of motion and resistance exercises. Persistent redness and swelling suggest inflammation, even if pain and tenderness cannot be felt because the area lacks sensation. If HO is found by radiological tests, medications are available to lessen the development of bone deposits in the muscles.

MUSCULOSKELETAL PAIN

During acute hospital care and early rehabilitation, upper extremity and shoulder pain are very common, but can be readily managed. At first, people with quadriplegia have more musculoskeletal pain than those with paraplegia. Poorer muscle strength in the arms predisposes to more pain in the joints, ligaments, and muscles of the neck, shoulders, and wrists. This can interfere with therapy and functional improvement. Neck pain and headache can accompany cervical and shoulder girdle muscle strain.

Musculoskeletal pain at the beginning of rehabilitation is a strong predictor for pain 1 year after in-patient rehabilitation, so medical efforts must be taken to manage this type of pain. Transfers and wheelchair mobility can lead gradually to overuse of the shoulders and wrists, causing pain. Any pre-injury arthritis or other joint problems can be exacerbated by the new demands that impaired strength and coordination make on the joints, especially in the knees of people who are recovering the ability to walk.

Treatments include range of motion and resistance exercises, anti-inflammatory medications, massage, analysis of how to make movements without exacerbating pain, and prevention of overuse of the affected part.

Spinal Nerve Root Pain

Trauma to the spinal cord often includes the nerve roots at the level of injury in cervical and thoracic injuries, and can affect several levels of roots in lesions below T11. The dorsal roots carry sensory information, including pain, which travel up the spinal cord to the brain. Trauma can cause pain signals to be generated in these roots, such as localized burning, electrical, and shooting pain.

Central Neuropathic Pain

Pain at and below the level of injury is common after SCI, even if there is no pain-generating pathology in the body. In these cases, the pain arises because of disordered connections among neurons in the pain pathways of the injured spinal cord. This type of pain is called *central neuropathic pain* (CNP) because it is generated by damage to the central nervous system. Touching the skin can cause the unpleasant feeling of tingling or burning. People with CNP describe many such sensations at rest, especially when trying to fall asleep. Patches of skin might feel hot or cold, or they might burn, tingle, ache or throb, or feel constricted or twisted.

CNP can arise from the intraspinal terminations of the nerve roots, or in the neurons of the dorsal horns of the spinal cord. Once these

> Pain at and below the level of injury is common after SCI, even if there is no pain-generating pathology in the body.

abnormal pain signals reach the brain, they influence how we perceive and respond to pain. The part of the brain called the *thalamus* modifies sensory input and processes the emotional components of how we perceive and respond to pain. In SCI, the usual processes that control the excitation and inhibition of electrical and chemical signals go awry, and the nervous system loses its ability to manage the thresholds for pain.

Pain can lessen the quality of a person's life more than any other consequence of SCI. CNP often starts soon after SCI. If it is delayed until several months after the initial injury, it might be due to an enlarging cystic channel within the cord, a syrinx, as discussed previously. Alternatively, it might not be pure CNP, and other inciting causes should be sought, such as slippage of nonfused bony vertebral bodies or other types of bodily injury that can increase spasticity and dysreflexia. Any ongoing, harmful sensory input to the cord, for example from a joint or the bladder, can exacerbate CNP. The source of CNP must be determined by physical examination, radiological studies, and laboratory tests.

Pain can be lessened with a variety of drugs such as anti-inflammatory agents and other analgesics, medications used for epilepsy such as carbamazepine and gabapentin, antidepressants such as tricyclics like amitriptyline (Elavil®) and selective serotonin reuptake inhibitors (SSRIs) such as fluoxetine (Prozac®), oral and intrathecal baclofen, clonidine or opiates, transcutaneous electrical stimulation, acupuncture, spinal cord and direct brain electrical stimulation, and rarely, surgical ablation of a pain pathway. Combinations of these approaches should be tried with patience and persistence.

SKIN BREAKDOWN

Any skin surface that is easily compressed against the inner bone—such as the back of the head, heels, hips, bottom of the spine (sacrum), and scapula—can become the site of irritation and redness. Layers of skin can be lost until eventually the muscle or bone is exposed and inflammation and infection develop. Pressure, or skin, ulcers (commonly called "bedsores") occur when friction, shearing, or compression of the skin lowers the blood flow to areas that already have compromised circulation because of autonomic impairment. Cellular damage follows. Additional predisposing factors to pressure sores include being underweight, poor nutrition, incontinence with persistently moist skin, poor alertness and memory that limits awareness of the need to monitor the skin, marked spasticity that puts joints and skin in abnormal postures, using pain medications that induce sleepiness, and smoking.

Prevention is far more effective than treating skin breakdown after it occurs. Minimize the possibility of bedsores with these preventative measures:

- Change position every 2 hours in order to take weight off bony surfaces; this is essential for people who cannot move in bed on their own.
- Use pillows and wedges to protect the skin in joint areas.
- Press against the arms of the wheelchair to lift the body and take weight off the buttocks; this should be done a few times an hour.

> Skin ulcers (bedsores) occur when friction, shearing, or compression of the skin lowers the blood flow to areas that already have compromised circulation because of autonomic impairment.

- Use proper padding of the bed and chair to avoid skin reddening, an early sign of skin breakdown.
- Use protection against sunburn, hot water, and hot surfaces as part of the daily routine, especially since the patient might lack the sensitivity to pain that would ordinarily alert them to danger.
- Limit pool exercise to avoid overly softening the skin or abrading it; lubricants can minimize friction and excessive drying of the skin.

If a pressure ulcer develops, care can include any of a variety of gels and protective film coverings, antibiotics, and surgical removal of infected and dead tissue. Healing can take months. The skin is never quite the same, however, once an open wound has healed. Future care of the area is especially important and must be done diligently.

SPASTICITY

Voluntary movement is controlled in part by signals from neurons in the cerebral cortex, whose axons descend in the corticospinal tracts (see Figure 1-4). These neurons are often referred to as *upper motor neurons*. SCI interrupts the corticospinal tracts and produces changes in muscle tone and reflexes below the level of injury. These changes are known collectively as *upper motor neuron syndrome* and include weakness or paralysis, fatigability, reduced dexterity and speed of movements, and an abnormality of muscle tone and reflexes called *spasticity*. This includes increased muscle tone (increased resistance to passive limb movement), hyperactive reflexes, involuntary rhythmic contractions of muscles that move a limb in a shaking motion called *clonus*, and spasms that flex or extend the legs, back, or arms.

Spasticity in the presence of severe weakness or paralysis can lead to stiffening of arm or leg muscles into abnormal postures, such as marked flexion of the arm or extension and crossing of the legs. Unmanaged, the combination of paralysis and severe increase in muscle tone can cause contractures of joints, which means the muscle tendons become permanently shortened and the muscles are unable to lengthen into a relaxed position. Increased muscle tone and spasms, however, do not have to be treated unless they interfere with joint range of motion or cause symptoms. For example, many people with SCI make use of their ability to induce leg flexion or extension spasms to aid in transfers or standing. Some enjoy the spontaneous movements and find that the high muscle tone increases the mass of their leg muscles. Many people have spasms only when they go from sitting to lying down, owing to stretch of the hip muscles. The brief clonus and extension of the legs otherwise does not interfere with sleep or wheelchair activities.

Shortening of muscles and tightening of joints can be prevented by moving each affected joint through its full range of motion several times a day using slow movements that are repeated about ten times. Putting weight through the joints of an arm or leg by leaning into an extended arm or standing up straight can briefly lessen muscle tone and the likelihood of developing contractures. Spasticity will increase in the presence of any negative stimulus, such as an infection or overfilling of the bladder, a rectal sore or fecal impaction, a pressure sore, an ingrown toe-nail, joint inflammation (arthritis), or tight-fitting clothing. These sources of irritation should be eliminated before trying medication.

Spasticity must be treated more aggressively if the spasms cause pain or interfere with sleep, wheelchair use, or transfers. Medications often help, but they can have side effects. Medications prescribed for spasticity include:

- **Baclofen:** 5–20 mg before sleep can lessen overnight spasms. From 5–40 mg, four times a day helps most people with spasms that recur all day. Baclofen must be tapered off slowly to avoid withdrawal seizures. Baclofen given intrathecally (pumped directly into the spinal fluid) improves the quality of life in patients who have been unable to control spasticity with oral medication.
- **Tizanidine:** 2–8 mg, up to four times a day can be helpful.
- **Clonidine:** up to 1 mg, three times a day is similar to tizanidine, but is more likely to lower blood pressure.
- **Benzodiazepines** such as clonazepam and other medications such as gabapentin and dantrolene can also lessen the frequency and severity of spasms.
- **Botulinum:** when just one or a few muscles have tightened from increased tone, an injection of botulinum toxin can relax them for a few months. The effect might last longer when combined with daily stretching and range of motion exercises with weight bearing through the affected joints.

Sometimes, antispasticity medications combined with physical therapy can improve coordination for reaching, grasping, or walking with weak but usable muscles. However, treating spasticity alone will not improve strength or coordination in paralyzed arms or legs.

SYRINGOMYELIA

The slit-like cavity inside the center of the spinal cord is called the *central canal*. It can expand even months or years after SCI if adhesions (scar tissue) are formed that tether the outer surface of the spinal cord to the overlying membranes, or if mechanical obstruction impedes the flow of spinal fluid within the central canal. The syrinx cavity enlarges up and down the cord from the original site of injury, following the path of least resistance and causing a condition called *syringomyelia* (Figure 4-2).

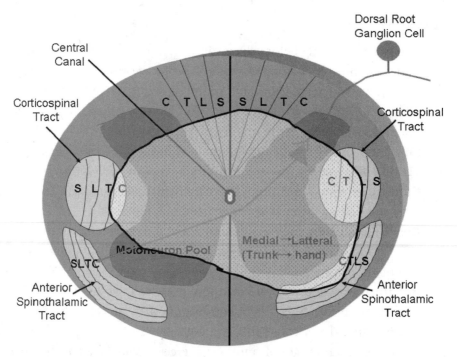

FIGURE 4-2

Syringomyelia. Enlargement of the central canal due to failure of proper spinal fluid flow following SCI can cause symptoms similar to those of an expanding mass such as a tumor within the spinal cord. This includes loss of temperature and pain sensation at the level of the syrinx due to interruption of sensory nerve fibers crossing the midline of the cord to enter the anterior spinothalamic tract, weakness and atrophy of muscles supplied by motor neurons at the level of the syrinx, and progressive weakness and loss of pain and temperature sensations spreading down from the level of the syrinx due to compression of the corticospinal tracts and anterior spinothalamic tracts from within. Because the syrinx can expand in an asymmetric (lopsided) way, the symptoms may be worse on one side of the body than the other, although the loss of pain and temperature sensation at the level of the syrinx is seen on both sides because those fibers cross the midline from both the right and left side just below the central canal. Bowel and bladder symptoms are also common.

Symptoms of syringomyelia include increased dysreflexia, CNP, further loss of sensation or movement, greater spasticity with more spasms, and additional bowel or bladder control problems. For more details, see the legend of Figure 4-2. Any worsening of these symptoms might require an MRI study of the spinal cord to look for syringomyelia. Surgery might be necessary to drain the fluid out of the syrinx and cut away the adhesions. A permanent catheter can be left in place to shunt the syrinx fluid into the abdomen, where it can more easily be absorbed into the blood.

SUMMARY OF TREATMENT OPTIONS

Prevention and management of the health-related complications of SCI require a commitment to long-term effort by the person with quadriplegia or paraplegia, by their caregivers or other people dear to them, and by a doctor with experience in neurologic diseases and their medical complications. Prevention necessitates a compulsively carried out set of routines for daily care that is derived from experience and solid information.

Persistent or worsening problems require early and thorough investigation to prevent a decline in health and function. Hospitalizations related to SCI arise mostly from making errors of omission and commission. Prevention takes time and energy, but the payoff is great. By reaching for a standard regimen of best care and building some reserve through fitness exercises, people with SCI have the opportunity to participate in all home and community activities.

> Prevention takes time and energy, but the payoff is great.

CHAPTER 5

What Happens During Rehabilitation?

THE GOALS OF NEUROLOGIC REHABILITATION include the prevention and management of acute and chronic medical complications, therapies to lessen impairments such as weakness and loss of feeling, teaching compensatory skills to lessen disability, training mobility and self-care skills, providing assistive devices, and reintegrating the person back into the home and work environment at the highest level of physical, psychological, and social functioning possible. This requires an interdisciplinary rehabilitation team approach.

After acute care, patients who are not able to walk and perform basic self-care independently usually go to an inpatient rehabilitation unit for training. The environment of these units is designed to lessen the anxieties associated with a new debilitating illness and the threats to functional independence. The team of doctors, nurses, and physical, occupational, speech, cognitive, and recreational therapists helps patients understand, articulate, and achieve short-term and longer-term goals that will improve their quality of life. Training procedures are structured to accommodate the present and changing capacities of patients.

Problem-solving skills become essential for every aspect of care, from bowel, bladder, and skin management to dressing, bathing, grooming, transferring from bed to wheelchair, and improving mobility. Therapists, patients, and families must collaborate in setting and revising goals and in carrying out therapies. In addition, changes in the home, such as making doorways wide enough for a wheelchair, installing ramps in place of stairs, and making countertops and sinks accessible, might have to be planned.

67

Very few specific therapies have been scientifically tested to determine if they work better than other approaches. Some people benefit from physical and occupational therapy strategies that do not help others. Gains depend on many factors, including the amount of voluntary movement and sensation, the spinal level and completeness of the injury, medical and physical problems that interfere with reaching best outcomes, prior athleticism, problem-solving skills, and willingness to make an effort. Small additional improvements can often be made in tasks that are practiced even years after SCI.

CHANGES IN IMPAIRMENT

Nearly all people regain some movement and sensation after SCI (Table 5-1). The baseline neurologic examination using the ASIA scales for grade, motor score, and sensation (see Figure 1-2) is not accurate until at least a few days after injury. Pain, medications, head trauma, and other factors tend to limit certainty as to whether a person is ASIA A or B, and whether they have some movement or sensation below the level of injury.

After the first few days, a spectrum of biological changes evolves. The patient's condition might improve as the negative impact of swelling,

Table 5-1 Conversion in ASIA Score over Time after Injury

	2-3 days after onset (percent of all acute SCI cases)	1 year after onset (percent that improve for each grade)
ASIA A	40-55	20 (B or C)
B	10-15	50 (C or D)
C	10-15	70 (D or E)
D	20-30	20 (reach E)
E	Not applicable	

This table shows that as time goes by, SCI patients tend to move from ASIA categories indicative of poor neurologic function to ones indicative better function. ASIA A = no movement or sensation below the level of injury; B = some sensation but no movement below the injury; C = some non-useful movement below the level of injury; D = useful movement but not normal below the level of injury; E = normal motor and sensory function below the level of injury.

bleeding, and inflammation resolve over several weeks, and as the ability of nerves to conduct electrical and chemical messages along spared descending and ascending pathways is restored. In addition, gene-driven

> Nearly all people regain some movement and sensation after SCI.

regenerative signals and other innate biological mechanisms can activate sprouting of collateral branches from preserved axons to connect to unaffected neurons within the spinal cord. This increases the number of spinal cord neurons that can respond to commands from the centers for motor control in the brain. Neurons that have lost their synaptic inputs can shrink (atrophy) and become electrically inactive, but still remain alive. If they are reinnervated by collateral sprouts of axons that were spared during SCI, these neurons can recover their function.

The brain also plays a growing role as movements are practiced. Clusters of neurons within the brain that are responsible for moving arm, hand, or leg muscle groups can adapt to help take over movements. For example, command signals that used to tell the wrist to extend can be trained to also assist the fingers to open and close. Thus, a prognosis for no further gains cannot be considered accurate for weeks and often months after SCI. For example, Table 5-1 reveals that people who are ASIA B or C at 72 hours after SCI have a 50–70 percent chance of achieving 1–2 level higher status by 6–12 months after their injury.

THE ZONE OF INJURY

Improvement in the ability to move is especially likely to be seen at the level of the injury and at least one level below, even after a complete SCI. These gains occur because there is a zone of partial preservation just outside the region of maximum damage. This zone of partial preservation can temporarily be neurologically silent but capable of resuming physiologic activity. Thus, there are sensory and motor levels below the recorded neurologic level that remain partially innervated and can

> Functional gains can be enhanced by
> practicing movements involving muscles
> above and within the zone of injury.

mediate partial recovery. The mechanisms underlying neurologic or functional improvement within this zone of injury can include:

- Short distance regeneration of injured axons
- Collateral sprouting of spared axons to reinnervate neurons that initially lost their synaptic input
- Collateral sprouts originating in the axons of spared motor neurons that reinnervate muscle fibers that have lost their motor neuron
- Short distance changes in descending axons from cerebral-controlling neurons for a specific muscle

Functional gains can be enhanced by practicing movements involving muscles above and within the zone of injury.

PARTIAL FUNCTION AS A PREDICTOR OF RECOVERY

Because of the mechanisms described above, it is clear that partial preservation of neurons and axons allows for the possibility of functional recovery. Any movement or sensation that is present below the level of the lesion during the first 4–8 weeks after SCI implies partial preservation of underlying neuronal structure and, therefore, the likelihood of additional movement and greater functional use of the arm or leg is high. Table 5-2 shows the average increase in strength by 1 year after injury in relationship to the initial ASIA grade of completeness of the injury. ASIA A subjects might only improve within the zone of partial preservation, whereas other groups tend to improve below this zone.

BUILDING MOTOR CONTROL

Motor control is a term that includes all the pathways and connections of the brain and spinal cord that can be called into play during training to

Table 5-2 Average Number of Points Gained on the ASIA Motor Scale at 1 Year after Cervical SCI (Figure 1-2)

Initial ASIA Grade	Motor Points Gained
A	10
B	30
C	40
D	30

This table reflects two contributing factors: the tendency for improvement to be greater in proportion to the more neural tissue that is preserved, and a ceiling effect when initial function is already close to normal.

make desired movements. Therapy to improve motor control takes many forms. When no movement is yet possible below the SCI, physical and occupational therapists can work with the patient on exercises to strengthen muscle groups, improve balance during sitting, reaching, and transfers, and teach ways to perform routine tasks needed for everyday activities. As small, new movements evolve, the therapists will build them into the components of additional movements.

For example, in Chapter 3, the patient in Figure 3-1 was able to flex his elbow, but not extend the wrist (cock the wrist back) or grasp objects in his hands after surgical fixation for his C5 incomplete SCI. Within days, he was able make a slight pinch of his thumb to the side of the second finger. With practice, he was able to pinch grapes and finger foods to put into his mouth. His therapists and family assisted by placing his hand and arm in the best positions to make successful movements for simple tasks. He practiced for 10–20 minutes, four times a day, making small movements, then larger ones at one joint, and then across several joints.

The skill with which he made this hand-to-mouth motion improved. By 4 weeks, he could fully feed himself, including cutting up foods, because his repetitive practice was associated with more finger flexion (bending) and wrist and elbow extension (cocking back the wrist and straightening the elbow), even though the muscles involved were still so weak that he was barely able to move these joints against gravity. If his arm was stretched out straight in front of him, he was barely able to cock his wrist back with his palm facing down. If his palm was facing up he was hardly able to bend his elbow so as to raise his hand.

Over the next 4 months, he became more independent in self-care as he practiced repetitively to improve speed, range, force, and accuracy of specific movements, such as those needed to grasp a cup, manipulate his clothing, hold a fork, cut up soft foods, and manage a catheter to empty his bladder. He learned to pre-shape his hand to the object he wished to grasp and coordinate more muscles across joints to reach and use light items. He repeated every movement again and again to make it more smooth and automatic.

PRACTICE LEADS TO LEARNING

Learning occurs when the connections between neurons (synapses) grow stronger from repetitive use. Practice might require the help of another person to set up items or to assist a goal-directed movement. Psychophysical and functional imaging studies show that during the performance of useful activities, many parts of the brain are active almost simultaneously. In order to be effective in improving performance, it is not sufficient to practice separately the simple movements of individual muscles involved in an activity. Practice must include performance of challenging and meaningful actions. For example, rather than simply trying to clasp the fingers, a person can recruit many regions of the brain to help reach for and grasp, and then release an item. Reaching for a cup and bringing it to the mouth to drink is an act the nervous system has been designed to perform—even a newborn can do this. It is also psychologically more meaningful than simply squeezing a ball. Thus, it is more apt to engage one's attention and the attention of the brain's interconnected controllers for actions.

Practices should vary. For example, a person can reach from different angles for items of different weights and diameters while sitting and, if possible, while standing. This continuous attempt to upgrade skills also poses new challenges for supporting the posture of the trunk. Strengthening exercises can accompany acquisition of skills by the arm and hand. Light hand or wrist weights, or elastic strips wound around the forearms or gripped with the fingers, can be used in sets of 10–15 repetitions to improve the strength of the different muscles that are brought into play when the angles of the movement are varied.

Biofeedback can be used to focus attention on the small number of voluntary muscles whose contractions can be controlled. With practice, these muscles can become activated more readily, and others recruited to increase the force or range of motion of a joint. Although strength can improve, there is little evidence that any type of biofeedback enhances functional use of the arm or hand by increasing the number of muscles that can be controlled voluntarily.

INCREASING FUNCTIONALITY THROUGH RECONSTRUCTIVE SURGERY

Reconstructive surgery aims to improve the independence of patients who have lost their arm or hand function due to cervical SCI. Surgical procedures include the following:

- Moving a muscle tendon from its normal insertion on bone to another place in order to alter movement
- Dividing or attaching a tendon to stabilize a joint
- Fusing a joint to eliminate motion
- Reshaping a bone

Tendon transfer procedures provide the potential to restore key functions, such as elbow or wrist extension, flexion of fingers, and finger pinch or hand grip control. Only experienced surgeons should be consulted regarding these sometimes delicate procedures.

Functional neuromuscular stimulation electrically activates a muscle to contract. By activating several muscles simultaneously, or in a rapid sequence, simple functional movements can be made. For example, The NeuroControl FreeHand System™ was developed for patients with C5 and C6 quadriplegia. Using this system, tiny wires are placed painlessly into eight muscles. These wires are controlled by a position sensor at the shoulder. A particular motion of the shoulder causes activation of muscles that produce wrist extension with either a pinching motion of the thumb against the side of the forefinger, as in grasping a key, or a larger grasping with the palm, as in holding a cup. Although this system

> Functional neuromuscular stimulation electrically activates a muscle to contract.

allowed considerably more use of the hand, its popularity was less than anticipated. The complexity, invasiveness, expense, and maintenance of any stimulator system can affect its acceptance by patients. Miniaturization, injectable electrodes such as the BION, and better computerized control systems that include sensory feedback to make force adjustments more accurately are all being studied.

Self-Care Skills

Self-care skills can be limited by the level and severity of the SCI, but often they can be reacquired with the help of assistive devices and good problem-solving skills. In general:

- If only C5 levels are intact, hand cuffs are needed for scooping food to the mouth, bladder catheterization requires assistance from another person, and an electric wheelchair is necessary. Typing at a computer can be performed with a mouthstick.
- With C6 intact for wrist extension, a cuff device can provide independent feeding and writing ability; driving is possible using hand controls.
- With C7 intact, feeding is independent, dressing becomes independent with assistive devices, self-catheterization is manageable, and a manual wheelchair can be operated.

Every retraining technique that aims to improve a motor skill, whether for the arms or legs, requires up to several hours of concentrated practice daily.

Adaptive devices make daily living activities much easier; for example:

- Velcro closures can replace hard to manipulate buttons.
- A suction holder can keep a sliding plate in place.
- A shower seat prevents falls.
- A raised toilet seat with nearby handrail or a sliding board can make transfers possible.
- Cell phones, the Internet, and computer-driven environmental controllers to open doors and turn appliances on and off allow for more independence.
- For quadriplegic patients, especially those on a ventilator, microswitches can be used to interface with any electronic device for environmental control and computer work.
- Lightweight wheelchairs that can be adapted for various impairments, surfaces and sports, battery-powered and power-assisted wheelchairs, and wheelchair-accessible vans allow worry-free mobility and social interactions.
- Orthotics made of molded plastic can be used to better position or stabilize the wrist, fingers, or ankle. They can also be dynamic. For example, when the wrist is angled so that the back of the hand is extended, the fingers of a weak hand tend to flex, which can enable light grasp or pinch. The Handmaster System™ (NESS Ltd.) is an external orthosis that fits over the wrist and forearm, and incorporates three surface electrodes to stimulate pinch and grasp. A start and stop button controls each movement.

MOBILITY AND WALKING

About one-half of the people with a recent SCI will not regain the ability to walk without physical assistance. The majority of these non-walkers have a lesion graded ASIA A or B at the time of injury (Table 5-3). Unfortunately, if no motor recovery has evolved in the legs of ASIA A and B subjects by 8 weeks after SCI to reclassify them as ASIA C, the outlook for recovery of voluntary walking is poor. Mobility training in the use of a wheelchair that is designed to meet a person's needs and abilities can give most people a remarkable level of independence in the home and community.

Table 5-3 Prognosis of SCI by Initial ASIA Score

Cervical central cord injury	80 percent
ASIA A	2 percent
ASIA B	40 percent
ASIA C	70 percent
ASIA D	90 percent

Approximate percentage of patients graded in the first 72 hours after SCI who recover at least short distance functional walking by 1 year after their injury. Cervical central cord injury refers to a non-penetrating, contusive injury as described in Chapter 2 and illustrated in Figure 2-1D.

Walking with a reciprocal left-right-left-right pattern of stepping—as opposed to swinging both legs together through crutches, as can by done by a paraplegic—is accomplished in patients who have enough strength in the legs to limit the energy cost of walking to an acceptable level. People who can flex at each hip so that the thigh rises against gravity, and the lower leg extends against at least gravity, have a good chance of

> Mobility training in the use of a wheelchair that is designed to meet a person's needs and abilities can give most people a remarkable level of independence in the home and community.

progressing from standing to taking steps in the parallel bars, and then walking with some bracing. Any sign of voluntary movement offers the strong possibility of additional movements with practice.

Eighty percent of people with a cervical central cord injury regain the ability to walk, but many of them walk slowly and stiffly because of limited motor control and severe spasticity. Anti-spasticity medications can improve the ability to walk by allowing greater hip flexion to swing each leg. The most important component in the recovery of walking, however, is the actual voluntary speed and strength of the movements needed to swing one leg while standing on the other.

During normal walking, the legs alternate bearing the body's weight and swinging forward to advance along the ground. The leg bearing the weight is said to be in the "stance" phase, while the leg swinging forward is said to be in the "swing" phase of walking. Some people find that if they concentrate on pushing the leg that is in stance into the ground as they flex the hip of the other leg to initiate its forward swing, they can improve the automaticity of swing. This timing maneuver draws upon some of the complex reflexes of the spinal cord and helps the person to concentrate on recruiting the muscles for one leg to stand and the opposite leg to swing.

Strengthening is especially important for the trunk and leg muscles. Several sets of resistance exercises, 10–15 repetitions each, should be performed each day. These can be incorporated into daily routines. For example, while seated in a chair, a person with some control but persistent weakness of the leg can perform this simple isometric exercise:

- Flex at the hip to lift the knee toward the chest
- Simultaneously, push downward with the hand over the top of the thigh
- Hold each up and down exertion for 5 seconds

Repeated practice of standing up and sitting down with less and less reliance on pushing off with the hands can be performed ten times during every commercial break on television.

For wheelchair users, a lot of practice must go into learning how to transfer from a bed, chair, or car seat into and out of the wheelchair. People with C6 intact can usually operate a wheelchair. If C7 is intact, transfers and mobility become easier. Most ASIA A-C patients start by using a sliding board to help them make transfers in and out of a wheelchair during inpatient rehabilitation. As upper body and arm strength improve, therapists can train patients to combine trunk control, hand and leg positioning, nose-over-toes forward lean, and timing in order to make successful transfers without the board. For some patients, a rigid neck collar, halo, or Thoraco-Lumbo-Sacral-Orthosis (TLSO; back brace) can prevent independent transfers until the bracing is removed.

Until learned skills become more automatic, it takes courage to do the first transfers, the first "wheelies" that lift the front wheels of the chair off the ground, the first independent ride on a downhill ramp, and the first trips out into the community.

Treadmill Training

The technique of treadmill training with partial body weight support (BWSTT) was developed based on studies of spinal cord circuits that have evolved to simplify rhythmical flexion and extension of the hind limbs of mammals for stepping. The technique has not enabled people to walk over ground if they have no motor control of their legs. However, by supporting people with incomplete SCI in a harness attached to an overhead lift, BWSTT can allow them to practice stepping with the manual assistance of a therapist in a way that optimizes their use of what motor control they possess.

A North American clinical trial of BWSTT was conducted with 145 people who were admitted for rehabilitation and were unable to walk. They received either BWSTT or conventional training for walking after an acute incomplete SCI. The subjects in each group were entered into the clinical trial within 8 weeks of SCI, at a time when they could not walk. They received training for 12 weeks. At 6 and 12 months after SCI, no differences were found between the two groups of patients in walking speed, walking distances, or need for assistive devices. Remarkably, the patients classified as ASIA B, C, and D who did walk were able to do so quite well. Over 90 percent of the subjects graded ASIA C and D on admission to the rehabilitation center in each group recovered. On average, they walked over ground (not on a treadmill) at a rate of nearly 2 miles per hour, wearing one ankle brace and using a cane for balance.

Robotic assistive devices such as the Lokomat™ have also been employed to improve training on a treadmill. These devices allow patients to place their feet into attached boots that are properly aligned, permitting them to engage in correct walking without the need for a therapist to guide their steps. To date, no studies have shown a better outcome than with more conventional training in parallel bars and over ground. Indeed, any form of treadmill training must be accompanied by practice over ground if walking is the goal. In addition, no studies have shown that any treadmill walking strategy in people who cannot step over ground will improve muscle or bone metabolism. More research is needed to test these types of training in patients who still walk poorly, or not at all, more than 6 months after SCI.

Other Mobility Aids

Passive standing in a frame that supports the legs can lessen leg spasms and help prevent orthostatic hypotension. However, no studies show that this improves bone or muscle mass. Some people can walk short distances using a knee-ankle-foot orthosis (KAFO; a brace that supports the leg from above the knee down to the foot), or a reciprocal gait orthosis that uses a mechanical cable system to control hip extension (straightening the hip as you do when you stand up from a sitting position) while assisting hip flexion (bending the hip as you do when you raise your knee toward your chest).

Functional neuromuscular stimulation devices have been developed over the past 30 years, but they have not achieved routine use. Stimulating as few as three muscles in each leg can assist an ASIA A or B paraplegic person to take steps on flat ground while supporting some body weight with the arms pressing into a walker (Parastep System™). Upper body strength and stamina must be quite good. Contraindications include bony fractures of the legs, osteoporosis, contractures, and impaired heart or lung function. Battery failure can lead to falls.

For people who have some motor control below the level of injury, electrical stimulators that activate the foot can aid flexion of the hip, knee, and ankle during the swing of the leg forward. Stimulation of the muscles of the buttocks and thigh can help stabilize stance on each leg. Walking speed can then increase modestly.

Hydrotherapy (pool training) has a long history of use in neurologic diseases, including SCI. Some people are able to stand with less support in water. Weak muscles can move better with the buoyancy offered by water. For people who have some motor control, exercises can be performed against the light resistance of water. However, there have been no studies showing that water therapy provides a clear advantage over other forms of physical therapy in terms of improving function.

Functional Nerve Stimulation (FNS) for exercise of the leg muscles can provide a modest fitness effect. Pumping the large muscles of the legs against resistance while pedaling for 20 minutes a day for 3–4 days

> Some people are able to stand with less support in water.

a week can increase muscle mass, cardiovascular fitness, and lower serum cholesterol. Arm crank exercise against resistance, weight lifting, and sustained wheelchair activities such as playing tennis or basketball also improve fitness (Table 5-4).

Table 5-4 Adapted Sports with Standardized Rules

Archery	Sailing
Basketball	Scuba
Canoeing	Snow and water skiing
Fencing	Power wheelchair soccer
Football	Softball
Hand crank bicycling	Swimming
Golf	Tennis
Road racing	Weightlifting
Quad rugby	

SEXUAL ACTIVITY AND FERTILITY

Sexual activity is possible and important for most people with SCI. In surveys, approximately 60–75 percent of women with paralysis engage in sexual intercourse, 50 percent in oral sex, 40 percent in manual stimulation, 25 percent in vibratory self-stimulation, and 10 percent in anal intercourse. Married women with SCI have expressed the same rate of satisfaction with sexual activities as people of the same age without SCI. Emptying the bladder immediately after intercourse can reduce the possibility of bladder infections. Fertility can be nearly normal. Term deliveries require close medical supervision, but are common. The onset of labor, however, might not be sensed when the injury is complete and above T8.

About 40 percent of men with quadriplegia, and 60 percent with paraplegia, engage in sexual intercourse. Producing an erection from a stimulating thought usually requires that some of the descending pathways from the brain to the S2–S4 level remain intact. However, as long as the neurons of S2–S4 that innervate the penis are present, a reflexive erection with physical stimulation is available to most men. The quality of an erection might not be optimal, and pregnancy rates for the partners of males run about 50 percent of that of people without paralysis. Medications can increase the venous filling of the sponge-like penis for erectile function. Orally taken drugs include the sildenafil-type class (Viagra®).

The medicated urethral system erection (MUSE) places a pellet of an erection-inducing drug such as alprostadil into the opening of the penis. Vacuum pumps, penile constriction rings, and surgically implanted penis-stiffening prostheses are all useful options. Great care must be taken not to injure the skin. Ejaculation rates run over 90 percent, although semen can be expelled toward the bladder rather than discharged from the penis (*retrograde ejaculation*). The motility of sperm might be lower than normal, further reducing fertility. If pregnancy in the partner is desired, sperm might need to be collected by non-intercourse methods, such as by vibration of the base of the penis or electrical stimulation through the rectum.

Limitations on sexual activity include pain, spasms or dysautonomia induced by intercourse and orgasm, incontinence, the effort necessary for preparation and positioning, and concerns about not feeling attractive or being able to satisfy the partner. Education might be needed about foreplay, reflex erections, vaginal lubrication, and use of drugs such as sildenafil.

VOCATIONAL REHABILITATION

Vocational rehabilitation programs offer vocational assessment, counseling, medical and assistive technologies for the workplace, and job placement. Although the available programs vary, federal and state vocational rehabilitation, state worker's compensation, the Department of Veterans Affairs, the Social Security Administration, and other systems all serve people with spinal cord injuries.

AGING

Beyond the first several years after a serious SCI, quality of life issues tend to take precedence over whether or not a person can walk. When surveyed, people with persistent paraplegia are more likely to be concerned about managing their bowels and bladder, controlling pain, and overcoming barriers to participation in sexual, social, employment, and leisure activities than they are to be concerned about walking.

Health maintenance remains a challenge. The loss of sensation that occurs with SCI can mask the usual symptoms of pain in the legs or abdomen that would ordinarily alert non-paralyzed people to the existence of infections, pressure sores, and even appendicitis. As people age, joint pains, heart disease, constipation or incontinence, and bladder and kidney problems can develop. Cancer of the bladder occurs more often in people with SCI who require a catheter than in able-bodied people. Weight gain and arthritis aggravate the overuse of ligaments and weak muscles, which can compromise the muscles and joints that are used to compensate for lost functioning. More physical assistance might be needed if fatigability and reduced mobility result.

At the same time, most routine medical maintenance should be no different than what is done for people at the same age without SCI. This includes preventative measures such as Pap smears, mammography, stool test for blood, colonoscopy, blood pressure and cholesterol checks, and flu vaccinations.

Life satisfaction might be most connected to a person's perception of their overall health, feelings of control over their lives, usual roles in work and family, leisure activities, and social support. These issues also contribute to how well a person copes with aging. Boredom, loneliness, lack of transportation, conflicts with attendants and family, and drug or tobacco abuse can also contribute to errors of omission and commission that lead to pressure sores, infections, and other preventable complications. Stress, a decline in health, and depression interact with each other. People with SCI, like anyone who ages with a disability, must be proactive in getting medical and psychological assistance as soon as they become aware a problem is developing.

SUMMARY

The aim of rehabilitation is to increase the ability of people to be as independent as possible and to participate in school, at work, with family, and in the community. Doctors and therapists can help people with SCI solve functional problems, adapt to new circumstances, and acquire additional skills. Repetitive practice is the basis for improvements in voluntary movement and function. Practice leads to adaptations within the parts of the nervous system that have been spared, and can induce biological mechanisms for learning and support of regeneration.

Improvements in daily activities and community reintegration can continue beyond the time of formal inpatient and outpatient rehabilitation, when reasonable goals are set and the necessary skills are practiced. It is also important to maintain a high level of physical reserve for daily activities and recreation, including cardiovascular fitness and muscular strength. It is also critical to maintain vigilance in preventing medical complications.

CHAPTER 6

Assistive Technologies

ASSISTIVE TECHNOLOGY SUPPORTS PEOPLE who are disabled in the enhancement of their mobility, daily self-care, community living, recreation, ability to learn, and employment. Simple tools are offered in home health care catalogues and Web sites such as www.rehabtool.com, or may be suggested by an occupational therapist. Some simple assistive devices include:

- Velcro straps and elastic laces to tie shoes
- Grabbers to extend the person's reach
- Grab bars strategically placed in a stall shower and by the toilet to help maneuvering in the bathroom
- Bowls and plates that stick to the table to help avoid accidental spillage
- Utensils that attach to the wrist
- Clothes that can be put on easily

Patients should feel free to tinker with equipment, such as that shown in Table 6-1, and modify it to their personal preferences; for example:

- Braces and orthoses evolve with needs and in relation to the amount of gain in sensation and movement.
- Wheelchair options and fittings should be tailored to body size, ability, and most typical daily use.
- Environmental remote controls allow management of lights, curtains, doors, timers, and appliances.

Some assistive devices are simple to add to the home and inexpensive; others are sophisticated and more costly to design and install, including:

Table 6-1 Sampling of Adaptive Aids

Eat	Utensil with thick or palm handle; cuff holder
	Dish or bowl with food guard, scoop, and suction holder; finger bowel
	Cup with no-spill cover, holder, and straw
Dress	Velcro closures on pants and shoes
	Button hook, pull zipper, and grabber
Bathe	Automatic water temperature control
	Shower seat and transfer bench
	Wash mitt, long handle brush/sponge, and handheld or low shower hose
	Rails and grab bars
Toilet	Raised seat, rails, and grab bars
	Room to maneuver wheelchair
	Commode
	Soap dispenser
Mobility	Ramp, stair lift, reduce architectural barriers
	Transfer devices–mobile or ceiling mounted
	Standing frame
	Wheelchair for daily use and recreation–manual, power assist, and powered
	Scooter
	Accessible car or van with lift, hand controls, wheelchair mounts or special seats
Everyday Items	One-handed devices, such as jar openers and cutting boards with pins
	Microwave oven
	Door knob extenders
	Grabbers with jaws
	Book holder with page turner
	Lazy Susan on low shelf
	Accessible basket, pack, and water dispenser for wheelchair
Communication	Cell phone with Web access and emergency connections, and Bluetooth or other ear and speaker connector
	Pre-set speaker phone dialer with switch for automatic calling
Computer	Typing aids to tap keys and hold/swing arms
	Voice recognition and synthesizer
	Special interfaces–infrared, optical sensors, voice, microswitch, touch screen controls for keyboard; adapted software

Environmental Controllers	Electronic interfaces for appliances, lights, door opening, security system, and emergency services
	Mobile and fixed robotic assistive devices
Recreation	Bicycle with hand pedals
	Mono-ski and accessible gym equipment
	Sports wheelchair
	Adapted fishing rod, pool cue, and knitting holders

Adapted from, B Dobkin, *The Clinical Science of Neurologic Rehabilitation*, Oxford University Press, 2003

- Equipment for video security, bath trolleys, and stairwell lifts
- Computers that are voice-activated or use other forms of no-hands control (see www.madentec.com), allowing access to e-mail and the Internet
- Communication via a PDA with cell phone and e-mail/Internet access to streamline social and work activities; also provides security in case a wheelchair or automobile breaks down

WALKERS AND CANES

Devices to assist in walking are designed to allow greater weight bearing by the arms, help take the load off one or both legs during stepping, and improve balance and lessen the risk of falling. Putting a lot of weight onto the arms, however, shifts the burden from the normally large, energy efficient leg muscles to the smaller shoulder and arm muscles. If too much arm loading is required, walking is likely to be slow and effortful. Assistive devices that can be used include:

- A four-wheel or wheel-less walker can shift body weight onto both arms.
- A single point or quad cane can assist the stance phase of the weak leg to help unload it. A cane can also provide balance when swinging the opposite leg forward.
- Electrical stimulation of one or more leg muscles can be timed to aid clearance of the foot during swing by reflexively inducing flexion to lift the weak leg; in this way, muscle tone can be greatly increased.

An ankle-foot orthosis can aid foot clearance as the leg swings forward and help stabilize the knee in stance. If one leg has little usable strength, a long leg brace across the knee and ankle (knee-ankle-foot orthosis, KAFO) can make it work like a strut, but swinging it forward takes much energy.

Hand Orthoses

If the hand is weak, simple splints can prevent flexing at the wrist by slightly extending the wrist and spreading or extending the fingers. With wrist extension supported by a hand splint, the fingers may be able to passively flex to hold items in a palmar or three-finger pinch. Swinging arm troughs can allow better positioning of the forearm and hand when proximal weakness interferes with hand use. These simple maneuvers may allow better use of the devices for the arm and hand (see Table 6-1). Splints with elastic bands and functional electrical stimulation can add both better positioning of joints and optimize muscle contractions to increase useful hand pinch or grasp. Trial and error approaches are necessary.

Wheelchairs

Wheelchair users have created a number of blogs and magazines that offer interesting observations and insights into using anything that will move you on land or sea (see (www.newmobility.com). A wheelchair prescription, however, is more mundane. It considers many factors, including:

- Safety
- Comfort
- Balance (this may change with practice)
- Type of transfers
- Dimensions necessary for trunk and thigh support
- Cushioning to add support and ease pressure points on skin
- Ease of transportability and propulsion
- Types of terrain encountered

- Durability
- Recreational use
- Cost

Wheelchair cushions vary in weight, thermal and pressure distribution, stability, the amount of shearing allowed, and comfort. Choices are often made by trial and error. During the first 2–6 months of rehabilitation, people with paraplegia learn how to balance their body's center of mass above and below the injury. As balance, arm strength, and confidence increase, fewer safety features such as anti-tip bars and heavy brakes are necessary.

It is best to start with an adjustable chair. Later, the axle can be moved a bit forward to increase maneuverability. As *pushrim biomechanics* improve (the ability to propel the wheelchair efficiently by pushing the wheel rims with the hands), people who are more athletic tend to strip down their chairs to lighten them. A solid frame that is not adjustable tends to be more durable (see Figure 6-1A–D). In addition to safety, cost may also be a tradeoff in performance. Lighter, more maneuverable chairs may use more exotic, expensive materials to maintain strength.

Manual wheelchair propulsion is not energy efficient, and can lead to repetitive strain injuries at the shoulders and wrists. Greater weight— of the chair and the individual—along with poor manual propulsion mechanics predisposes individuals to injury. A propulsion stroke in which the hands drop below the pushrim appears to lessen the number of strokes by producing a greater push angle. Sitting too low or behind the wheels, also contributes to wrist injuries such as carpal tunnel syndrome. Excessive vibration of the chair can lead to back and other injuries. Ultralight wheelchairs have been shown to be more comfortable, ergonomically superior, and generally sturdier, than lightweight chairs. Unfortunately, it may be necessary to argue about this difference with Durable Medical Equipment insurance company providers.

The use of hybrid pushrim-activated, power-assisted wheelchairs is increasing. A motor in each wheel hub amplifies the push on the rim to assist on difficult terrain, carpets, and slopes. The wheels are removable for transport, which is necessary because they are too heavy to lift.

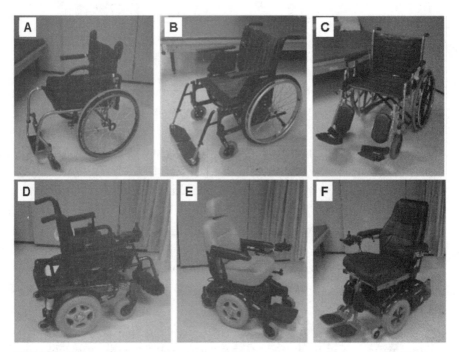

FIGURE 6-1

Wheelchair designs. A–C are manual wheelchairs; D–F are electric-powered wheelchairs.
(A) Ultralight, **(B)** lightweight, **(C)** and depot manual wheelchairs. Light weight and maneuverability are traded off against stability and adjustability. **(D)** Rearwheel, **(E)** midwheel, **(F)** and frontwheel drive electric-powered wheelchairs. As the drive-power wheel is shifted forward, maneuverability increases because the turning radius decreases, but control decreases due to fishtailing. Adapted from Cooper RA, Cooper R and Boninger ML, Wheelchair design and seating technology. In: Selzer ME, Cohen LG, Gage FH, Clarke S, Duncan PW, eds, *Textbook of Neural Repair and Rehabilitation*, Cambridge University Press, 2006.

Better actuator technology should lead to lighter and even more maneuverable systems.

A power wheelchair with heavy batteries underneath it can be remarkably maneuverable. They come in rear, mid, and front wheel drive models (Figure 6-1D–F), and primarily indoor (smaller base) and mixed use designs. Electromechanical brakes and fine-tuned controllers make them rather safe on even ground. However, safety can be compromised when going over a curb with a 45-degree tilt or descending a greater than 5-degree slope.

The front wheel power base is perhaps the most maneuverable, but it can fishtail on uneven ground. The controls come in flexible choices, including: joy sticks, chin pressure, sip and puff mouthpiece, and even voice command. Sensory and cognitive impairments, and spasms or movement disorders, will lessen their safe use. Batteries come in at least three sizes of increasing power storage (22, 24, and 27 groupings). Lead acid batteries are the least expensive; gel and absorbent glass mat batteries require no maintenance and are more durable.

The Independence 3000 robotic wheelchair or "IBOT" can rise to allow eye level contact with others, and adds the ability to climb steps using gyroscopes and a clever four-wheel base (Figure 6-2). This type of wheelchair is quite expensive. Table 6-2 lists the various options to be evaluated in a wheelchair prescription.

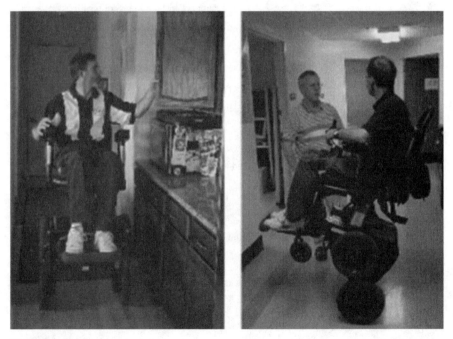

FIGURE 6-2

The IBOT. This expensive motorized wheelchair can elevate and balance on its hind-wheels. Adapted from Cooper RA, Cooper R and Boninger ML, Wheelchair design and seating technology. In: Selzer ME, Cohen LG, Gage FH, Clarke S, Duncan PW, eds, *Textbook of Neural Repair and Rehabilitation*, Cambridge University Press, 2006.

Table 6-2 Wheelchair Prescription Considerations

Frame	Weight
Seat	Height: needs to fit under a table; elbows at 90-120 degrees when hands at top of pushrim
	Width: an inch at most between each side and the trochanter
	Depth: sit with about 2 inches between front edge to back of knee
	Angle: 5 degrees or more of posterior tilt
	Footrest: fixed, removable, swing away, individual vs. bar, foot straps; leg at 70-95 degrees
	Cushion: foam, air, gel, fluid
	Clothing guards
	Inserts
Back	Angle: fixed at 90-100 degrees, or reclining back
	Height: support without interfering with use of arms
	Head rest for high quadriplegia
Arms	Height: fixed or adjustable
	Fixed, removable, table attachment
	Power control type and placement
Wheels	Material
	Rear axle: best if close to center of body mass
	Angulation: greater cam angle for sports
	Hand rims: ergonomic types
	Tires: width (weight of chair and riding surface), tread, pneumatic, or solid
Front Casters	Smaller diameter means greater rear wheel balance needed
Back Anti-Tip Bars	
Brakes	Locking, backslide
Power Supply and Controls	
Horns, Baskets, Pouches, Holders	

CHAPTER 7

Research to Find New Treatments for SCI

T HE GOALS OF ADVANCED RESEARCH into the treatment of SCI are three-fold:

1. The spinal cord is exquisitely sensitive to the cascade of biochemical events that magnify the impact of an injury, and researchers must discover ways to limit the damage to nerve cells and nerve fibers.
2. Lost nerve cells must be replaced, and interrupted axons must be encouraged to regenerate.
3. Restored anatomic connections must result in recovered function.

This chapter and Chapters 8 and 9 explore the cutting edge of SCI research in order to educate patients and their loved ones in assessing the treatments discussed in the media, which advances look promising, and whether to participate in a given clinical trial. Details regarding particular clinical trials have not been included, such as who is conducting them, whom to contact in order to participate, and who is eligible to enroll. By the time this book is published, the trials might have been completed, recruitment of patients could be over, or the trial might have been abandoned, making these details no longer relevant.

These chapters focus on the general principles involved in testing therapies for SCI, the mechanisms of damage to the spinal cord, and the scientific principles underlying the therapeutic approaches currently under consideration. There are many clinical studies relevant to SCI; most of them involve incremental advances in patient care. These studies are not discussed here; rather, the focus is on the clinical trials aimed at the most fundamental elements in preventing or reversing SCI.

Resource materials can be found at the end of this book, including advocacy organizations and Internet sites where up-to-date information can be obtained about the status of particular clinical trials. The information covered in the next three chapters is aimed at assisting interested readers in understanding the material that can be found on the Internet, in print media, and in newsletters.

The Stages of Research Trials

Before a drug treatment for SCI can be adopted for use in humans, a lengthy testing process takes place over many years. Although each

> Before a drug treatment for SCI can be adopted for use in humans, a lengthy testing process takes place over many years.

potential treatment is different, the typical sequence of events for an experimental drug is as follows:

(1) **Tissue Cultures.** Based on its chemical structure or similarity to other drugs, a chemical compound is predicted to have a neuroprotective or a regenerative effect, and it is tested on neurons in tissue culture in the laboratory. If it works in tissue culture, the results are published in a scientific journal after rigorous review of the manuscript by experts before acceptance for publication.

(2) **Animal Testing.** The drug is then tested in an animal model of SCI. For convenience, rats are usually used. If it is a naturally-occurring constituent of the spinal cord, such as a neurotrophic factor, mice that are genetically engineered to lack or have an excess of the tested substance are used. If the result is strongly positive, the study is published in a scientific journal. Usually, other scientists become intrigued and try the drug in their own experimental model. If the results are again positive, they publish additional articles.

(3) **Phase I.** Ideally, the next step is to test the drug on a non-human primate, such as a monkey. However, because such studies are very

expensive, in many cases, this step is skipped and the drug is tested on a small number of human patients in what is called a *Phase I* clinical trial. This is aimed at determining whether the drug is too toxic to use on humans, and to get some information about what a reasonable dose would be. Patients are given the drug at an estimated dosage that is determined by animal studies.

Physical exams, blood tests, and other types of observation are conducted, comparing the patients receiving the drug with those receiving a placebo, or "dummy" treatment, which is included in the experiment to control for the psychological effects of believing they are receiving a beneficial medication.

Double-blind means that the patients and the investigator do not know which patients are receiving the test drug and which the placebo. This is the best experimental design because it allows for the possibility that the experimenter might succumb to bias in interpreting the results, or might bias the patient by hinting at the expected outcome.

The number of patients in Phase I trials (20–80) is too small to give significant information about efficacy. Because they are not aimed at determining effectiveness, many Phase I clinical trials are open label (no placebo is used), especially if the mode of therapy is complex or unconventional, such as injections of antibodies into the spinal fluid or transplantation of cells into the spinal cord.

In Phase I trials, all the recruited patients are given the treatment and tests are performed to look for toxicity. The results are compared with standard historical data for similar groups of people in the community, and an estimate is made as to whether the treatment results in more side effects, such as liver or kidney damage, than would be expected for the general population.

(4) **Phase II.** If the drug (or other treatment) passes a Phase I trial, it goes to a somewhat larger clinical trial, *Phase II*, which might include 100–300 patients. The purpose of a Phase II trial is to determine the best dose by comparing two or more doses against each other and against placebo, and to obtain preliminary information on feasibility and efficacy of the treatment—this is called *proof of principle*.

Therefore, Phase II clinical trials should be prospective, randomized and controlled (defined below).

If a Phase II clinical trial does not suggest a significant beneficial effect, development of the drug or treatment generally stops. If the Phase II trial suggests that the treatment is effective, then a large scale *Phase III* clinical trial with hundreds or even thousands of patients is undertaken.

(5) **Phase III.** The "gold standard" of human therapeutic drug development is the Phase III, randomized, prospective, double blind, placebo-controlled, multicenter clinical trial (RPCT). *Randomized* means that as patients are entered into the trial, they are assigned randomly to receive the test drug at a particular dose or the placebo. This avoids bias in assigning patients to one or another part of the study. For example, if we know that less severely injured patients recover better than those with more complete injuries the researcher might assign patients with slightly less complete injuries to the test drug part of the study. Long experience has taught researchers that bias can be introduced subconsciously into an experiment, even in a large, well organized clinical trial and even by the most scrupulously honest investigators. This is not necessarily the result of an intention to cheat.

Prospective means that patients are entered into the clinical trial only after the trial has been designed and the ground rules agreed upon, rather than the researcher collecting information from the records of patients who were treated previously and trying to interpret the results according to criteria that make sense after the fact.

In most cases, approval of a drug by the U.S. Food and Drug Administration (FDA) requires that the efficacy of the drug be demonstrated in at least two Phase III clinical trials. The experimental protocol and statistical methods by which the data will be analyzed are negotiated in advance between the drug company and the FDA. The conduct of a Phase III clinical trial is usually monitored by an external panel of experts to be sure it is run correctly. If all this sounds like it must be very expensive, you are right. Most of the drugs that are tested never make it all the way to FDA approval, and the average cost to bring a new drug to market is currently more than $800 million, with the cost of Phase III trials being the largest expense.

Why Phase III Clinical Trials Are Necessary, Even When a Phase II Trial Shows Benefits

Considering how costly it is to do a Phase III study, and since the analysis of a Phase II clinical trial might result in a conclusion that patients given the test drug had an outcome that was statistically significantly better than those given the placebo, why is it necessary to do an even larger study?

There are several reasons. First, it is not possible to control for all of the variables that might affect the outcome. In addition, the smaller the trial, the fewer the variables that can be controlled. Therefore, a larger study allows the subjects to be categorized by age, sex, race, weight, and other factors, depending on what seems to be relevant, and to detect differences in drug effectiveness that might appear between these groups. Moreover, a larger size sample, if it is truly prospectively randomized, allows researchers to have more confidence that factors that were not actively controlled for because they had not been considered, would nevertheless be cancelled out. Larger samples also allow a greater chance of detecting serious but uncommon side effects that could be disqualifying, or at least point to laboratory tests that should be done in monitoring patients receiving a drug.

Finally, there is a hidden statistical problem that stems from the way small clinical trials are organized and reported. Let us assume that for a drug to be accepted as effective, statistical analysis must show that the probability (p) that the difference in effectiveness observed between the test drug and placebo could have occurred by random chance is no more than 5 percent. That is, if the test drug were really no more effective than placebo, and the clinical trial was repeated many times, the observed outcome would occur only once in twenty clinical trials. The statistical shorthand for this is that p is less than 0.05 (or, $p < 0.05$), which is a commonly used level of statistical significance applied as a criterion for accepting a conclusion in clinical and other biological research.

Scientists are free to start a clinical trial as long as they get permission from their local institutional review board (IRB), which certifies that the study is being done ethically and correctly. Suppose that five different groups of investigators decided to test the same drug, and only one of the groups got a positive result. This would effectively reduce the probability that the result could have occurred by random chance from one in twenty to five in twenty; for example that is $p < 0.250$, which would not be considered statistically significant. The four groups whose clinical trial was negative might never even publish their results, because there is no shortage of ineffective treatments and many journals would not be interested in publishing such a study. It would be difficult for anyone to know the real significance of the findings of a clinical trial, because they could not be sure how many times the study was done with opposite results.

> Scientists are free to start a clinical trial as long as they get permission from their local institutional review board (IRB), which certifies that the study is being done ethically and correctly.

To put it in a more cynical way, if someone wanted to trick the public into thinking that they had an effective treatment for SCI, they could repeat a small clinical trial over and over, until one of the trials gave a "statistically significant" positive result. The Phase III multicenter clinical trial can be more accurate. These trials are highly publicized in advance, have a protocol that is agreed upon by the FDA, and the outcome will be widely acknowledged to represent the best estimate of the effectiveness of the treatment. Moreover, because a Phase III trial is so expensive, it will not be undertaken lightly. If a second Phase III trial is required for FDA approval of a treatment and the trial results are positive, the public will likely have great confidence in the treatment. Even so, as we have seen with methylprednisolone, the results of a Phase III trial can sometimes be questioned.

WHO SHOULD PARTICIPATE IN A CLINICAL TRIAL?

Because SCI often imposes severe limitations on function and quality of life, it is understandable that patients and their loved ones feel a sense of desperation and might be willing to try almost anything in order to have a possibility of improvement. Even if the chances of improvement as a result of a clinical trial are slim, many patients develop a sense of mission and commitment to research that targets their medical condition. They want to make a valuable contribution to science, and to the ultimate discovery of a cure. They gain a sense of altruistic satisfaction by participating in research, even if it involves personal sacrifice. This is admirable, and it probably accounts for more participation in clinical trials than the expectation of personal benefit. But there can be something to lose. The possible complications of clinical trials include:

- Further worsening of neurologic function
- The development of painful conditions
- Infections
- Toxic effects on important organs such as the liver and kidneys
- Serious allergic reactions that can also damage organs
- In rare cases, even death

A poorly designed study based on inadequate scientific rationale is unlikely to provide the sort of valuable scientific data that the patient is hoping to contribute. Therefore, it is important that patients exercise judgment in deciding whether to participate in a given clinical trial. In order to help with this type of decision, a group of scientists has formed using the name "The International Campaign for Cures of Spinal Cord Injury Paralysis" (ICCP). This group is sponsored by several of the leading patient advocacy organizations in the field of SCI, and has been developing guidelines for the conduct of clinical trials in SCI.

The ICCP has put together a pamphlet, *Experimental Treatments for Spinal Cord Injury: What You Should Know*, which contains recommendations for patients to help them decide whether a given clinical trial is worthy of their participation. The recommendations include questions that patients should ask their doctor before agreeing to participate. These questions are organized into seven categories, together with the preferred answers, as follows:

Category #1

Are there safety risks associated with this experimental treatment?

Answer: Should be YES; no one can guarantee total safety.

Could my condition or my health get worse after this experimental treatment?

Answer: Should also be YES; if someone states there are little or no risks you should be wary.

If so, describe the possible risks associated with this experimental treatment.

Answer: The investigator should be able to discuss in detail the possible risks associated with any particular human study.

Category #2

What are the likely benefits of this experimental treatment?

Answer: The investigator should describe a range of possible benefits from very subtle to modest functional improvements.

What is the maximum level of recovery I might experience after this treatment?

Answer: Anyone who claims you are going to make a dramatic recovery with the return of almost full function should be avoided, because there is no evidence for any treatment of SCI having such striking outcomes.

How will any potential benefit be measured?

Answer: The investigator should be able to describe a number of different measures that will be used to evaluate your progress after treatment.

Is this outcome measure accurate and sensitive as a tool?

> **Answer:** The investigator should be able to describe the strengths and limitations of the evaluation procedures; once again, nothing is perfect.

Category #3

What is the preclinical evidence that this experimental treatment has benefit; for example, in animals with SCI?

> **Answer:** The investigator should be able to outline the evidence, including the strengths and limitations of the treatment approach.

Have these findings been independently replicated?

> **Answer:** This could go either way, but there should be evidence that other scientists have obtained similar results when investigating this therapeutic target.

If so, is there a consensus among the scientists that this treatment addresses a valid therapeutic target for improving functional outcomes? Are there any dissenting opinions, and do these arguments have some validity for not going forward with this treatment?

> **Answers:** The investigator should be able to provide you with a summary of the pros and cons for the treatment. If not, be wary of any treatment that is claimed to have no detractors; scientists are usually quite tough on each other. Use the Internet to look up the most recent publications on the proposed treatment. By this time, you will have learned enough basic biology and medicine to be able to understand most of what is written in any relevant scientific paper.

Category #4

Is this human study registered as a clinical trial with an appropriate, qualified regulatory body?

Answer: Should be YES, and the investigator should be able to provide you with details immediately. If the answer is vague on this point, you should be wary.

What phase in the clinical trial program is this particular human study (Phase I, Phase II, or Phase III)?

Answer: Should be immediate and in as much detail as you want.

Is there a control group in this study?

Answer: Should be YES. If NO, this should be a Phase I study. If not Phase I, the human study is unlikely to be a clinical trial and you should be wary.

Could I be randomly assigned to the control group?

Answer: Should be YES. If NO, this is likely not a valid clinical trial.

For how long after the treatment will I be assessed for a change in my functional outcome?

Answer: Should be anywhere from a minimum of 6 months to a year after treatment.

Will I know whether I have received the experimental or the control treatment?

Answer: If at all physically possible, the answer should be NO. If YES, it should be a Phase I trial. If not a Phase I, you should be wary that this is not a valid clinical trial. Sometimes you cannot help but know what group you are in, but you should be asked not to disclose to the examiners whether you are in the experimental or control group.

Will the investigators and examiners be blind as to what treatment I have received?

Answer: This should be a definite YES, unless it is a Phase I trial. If NO, it is not a valid clinical trial and you should be wary.

Category #5

Will my participation in this clinical trial limit my participation in other SCI clinical trials?

Answer: Should be YES, this is a possibility.

If so, what types of trials am I likely to be excluded from in the future and for how long?

Answer: The investigator should be able to immediately outline which type of trials you might be excluded from in the future.

Category #6

Do I have to pay for treatment?

Answer: This should be NO. If YES, this is not a valid clinical trial and you should be wary.

Are there any other costs associated with my participation in this study?

Answer: Should be NO, other than the time and effort it requires to comply with the protocol.

Will my expenses associated with participating in this study be paid; for example, travel to a medical center for follow-up assessment?

Answer: Should be YES.

Category #7

Can you provide me with the names of several scientists and clinicians (not involved with this study) who can provide me with independent advice about this treatment and your reputation?

Answer: Should be YES, and you should be able to verify the credibility of the study and the credentials of the investigators easily and readily via the Internet.

The authors of this book agree with these questions and answers, and recommend that patients *avoid* unconventional treatments that are not part of a legitimate clinical trial.

CHAPTER 8

Research on Minimizing Damage to the Spinal Cord Immediately After Injury

T HE FIRST GOAL OF RESEARCH is to discover ways to limit the damage to nerve cells and nerve fibers. This is called *neuroprotection*. Fortunately, in most cases of SCI, there is a delay between the impact causing the injury and the death of nerve tissue. This is because most cases of SCI do not involve penetration of the spinal canal by a missile or bone fragment—the injury is usually the result of a concussion. The spinal cord is slammed against the boney wall of the spinal canal as the result of a fall or other blunt trauma. If you could look at the spinal cord with a microscope immediately after an impact, it would appear normal. Hemorrhage and cell death develop over a period of hours, days, and sometimes weeks.

> The first goal of research is to discover ways to limit the damage to nerve cells and nerve fibers. This is called *neuroprotection.*

This gives us a "window of opportunity" to intervene with medications and other treatments. Therefore, a great deal of research is directed at determining the mechanisms of delayed neuronal death and axonal disruption, and discovering treatments that could prevent damage. Until now, only one treatment, intravenous methylprednisolone, has been accepted as effective in minimizing this delayed damage, although after reviewing the data, some experts think the evidence is shakier than believed at first. Nevertheless, methylprednisolone is administered routinely on the first day of hospitalization. However, several other approaches to neuroprotection are under intense study. Some of them have even gotten to the stage of human clinical trials.

How Nerve Cells Die

Nerve cells have two main paths to cell death, necrosis and apoptosis (pronounced ay-pot-ohsis) (Figure 8-1).

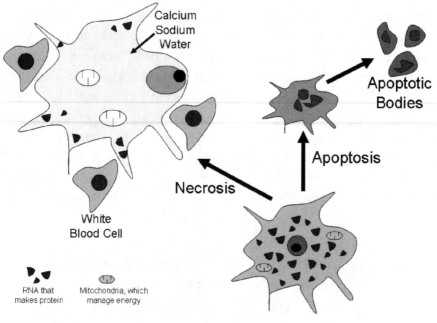

FIGURE 8-1

Death of Neurons in SCI Occurs by Mechanisms that Fall on a Continuum Between Necrosis and Apoptosis. Although classical pathology has characterized neuronal death as either necrotic (pathological), in which the cell blows up from loss of energy and membrane integrity, or apoptotic (spontaneous), in which the cell undergoes an orderly programmed dismantling, most cell death, including that occurring in SCI, involves mechanisms of both pure types (see text).

Necrosis

At one time, it was thought that all cells die in the same way. An injury occurs, such as trauma, poisoning, or loss of oxygen as in a stroke, causing the cell membrane to lose its integrity. Sodium and water leak into the cell, causing it to swell. Calcium also leaks into the cell, resulting in several toxic actions, including activation of calcium-dependent enzymes that digest the large fatty molecules making up the membranes and internal structures of the cell; for example, the *mitochondria*, which are the power plants of the cell that manage the storage and use of energy.

Some of the by-products of the calcium-activated, enzymatic digestion of fats in the cell result in the generation of toxic molecules called *oxygen free radicals*. These fat derivatives are exceptionally active in burning up (oxidizing) large molecules, which contributes powerfully to the disintegration of the neuron. The nucleus, mitochondria, and other internal structures also swell and can burst. The granules of RNA that make protein degenerate or move out of the cell body into the dendrites, and production of protein and other large molecules, stops. Soon the cell's contents leak out and the cell is not able to make the constituents that it normally makes to maintain its structure and perform its functions.

As the cell deteriorates, the debris causes inflammation. The white blood cells (*macrophages*) and the central nervous system's own immunological cells (*microglia*) are attracted to the area to ingest the cell debris. Blood flow to the area also increases, which, in turn, increases the rate of this "mopping up" process. This type of cell death is referred to as *pathological cell death* or *necrosis*.

The inflammatory response can also add to the damage through the release of cytokines by macrophages and white blood cells. Cytokines are molecules that are similar to neurotrophic molecules in that they bind to specific receptors on neurons and induce complicated biochemical effects in the cell. Some of these cytokines are beneficial in the regeneration of axons, but some cytokines are toxic to neurons and can cause even more cell death.

Apoptosis

More than 100 years ago, a second form of cell death, *spontaneous cell death*, or *apoptosis* was identified. In apoptosis—a process that can take days, weeks, or even longer—something activates "cell death programming" inside the neuron. Unlike necrosis, which requires no energy and is brought about by the loss of energy to the cell, apoptosis is an active process that requires energy and involves the synthesis of enzymes that participate in an orderly dismantling of the cell that includes:

- Chopping the genetic material (DNA) into regular-sized pieces
- Dividing up the nucleus into smaller particles
- Bundling the cell contents into smaller membrane-bound bodies (*apoptotic* bodies)
- Scavenger cells of the nervous system, the microglia, ingest the apoptotic bodies without triggering a full blown inflammatory reaction

A classic example of apoptosis can be seen during the development of most parts of the central nervous system. Initially, embryos have about twice as many neurons as they will ultimately have after birth. These neurons send out axons to make synapses with appropriate target cells, such as other neurons in the central nervous system—or muscle fibers in the case of motor neurons. These target cells provide small quantities of important proteins called *neurotrophic factors*, which are needed to maintain the health of the neuron.

Neurotrophic factors are manufactured in the target cells; then they move backwards across the synapse into the axon, where they are transported back to the neuron's cell body and are involved in a number of important biochemical processes. Because the target cells can only accommodate a limited number of synapses, the developing axons are in competition with each other for access to these targets. The neurons that fail to make a synapse are deprived of the target-derived neurotrophic factors and eventually die by apoptosis. Similarly, when SCI severs axons, the neurons lose their connections to the targets they depend on to supply them with neurotrophic factors and they can shrink (atrophy) or even die.

Many different neurotrophic factors have now been discovered, and it is believed that each neuron requires its own unique combination of neurotrophic factors. An attempt to gain knowledge about the large variety of neurotrophic factors in the nervous system, and the specific neurotrophic requirements of different classes of neurons, has been an important aspect of modern research in the treatment of SCI, traumatic brain injury, stroke, and other neurologic disorders.

The Reality of Cell Death

As interesting as this dichotomy between necrosis and apoptosis might be, in recent years it has been recognized that these processes rarely occur in their pure form, and that most instances of neuronal death involve a combination of molecular events that represent features of both necrosis and apoptosis. Nevertheless, the recognition that neurons rarely die instantaneously, but die in a delayed fashion involving complicated, active biochemical processes, has led to research on methods of neuroprotection, whereby therapeutic interventions during the delay between injury and neuronal death can save neurons and improve the ultimate ability to function after SCI.

Axon Interruption is also Delayed

Just as neurons do not die instantly in a concussion, so axons that are not severed by a missile or bone fragment might be stretched. They look normal when viewed with a microscope immediately after SCI. However, the stretch injury results in delayed damage, much of it apparently as a result of leakage of calcium into the axon and activation of calcium-dependent enzymes that over a period of about 8 hours disrupt the internal protein skeleton of the axon, leading to its severance.

EXPERIMENTAL NEUROPROTECTIVE THERAPIES

Several approaches have been devised to inhibit the mechanisms of cell death and axon disruption.

> Several approaches have been devised to inhibit the mechanisms of cell death and axon disruption.

Inhibitors of Oxygen Free Radicals and Anti-Inflammatory Drugs

A large number of neuroprotective strategies have been reported to improve the outcome of SCI in experimental animals. Unfortunately, this does not guarantee they will work in humans. For example, many of the same neuroprotective strategies were tested in patients with stroke after animal studies predicted they would reduce neural damage and promote recovery. Yet to date, none of these clinical trials have been successful.

NXY 059
The Astra Zeneca drug NXY 059, (an oxygen free radical "scavenger" that inactivates oxygen free radicals) showed great promise in animal studies. One Phase III clinical trial suggested that it had a favorable impact on overall disability, although it did not appear to alter the specific neurologic impairments that were a consequence of the stroke. The results of this trial were published in the *New England Journal of Medicine*, a prestigious medical journal. A second Phase III clinical trial of NXY 059, however, failed to demonstrate effectiveness, and development of this drug has stalled. There has been no clinical trial of NXY 059 for SCI.

GM1-ganglioside
A drug that inhibits the production of oxygen free radicals, GM1-ganglioside (Sygen®), was expected to promote recovery, but it failed to help people with SCI. GM1 also failed to help people with stroke. This does not mean that *no* oxygen free radical scavenger will prove effective for SCI.

Methylprednisolone
As discussed previously, methylprednisolone, a corticosteroid drug, has long been used to suppress the immunological component of the neuronal damage in SCI. Yet clinical trials failed to show evidence of improved

outcome. It was only after the dose was increased to far above the immunosuppressive levels that several multicenter clinical trials (NASCIS 1, 2 and 3 in the U.S., and a study in Japan) showed evidence for improvement in neurologic outcome, although the magnitude of the benefit was relatively small.

It is suspected that the mechanism underlying high dose methylprednisolone effectiveness is inhibition of oxygen free radical production. Even these results are now being reconsidered based on details of data analysis, and on the results in other studies that are less positive. The NASCIS 2 and 3 studies included investigation of two other drugs that had been found to be neuroprotective in animals:

- Naloxone (NASCIS 2 and 3), an inhibitor of the opioid receptors that mediate of the effects of narcotics and endogenous morphine-like molecules (endorphins) on neurons
- Tirilazad (NASCIS 3), a synthetic corticosteroid that has fewer toxic properties than methylprednisolone

Both of these drugs appeared to be less effective than methylprednisolone, and whether they have any significant neuroprotective benefit is still controversial.

TRH

A promising drug that showed neuroprotective effects in animals is *thyrotropin releasing hormone* (TRH), a hormone which is released by the pituitary gland and stimulates the thyroid gland to release thyroid hormone. Like naloxone, TRH inhibits the effects of endorphins that are released in the spinal cord at the time of injury. In a very small trial (20 patients) conducted in the U.S. and published in 1995, TRH treatment appeared to be associated with a better outcome than placebo, although only for incomplete SCI patients. This suggested that it would be worthwhile to do a large scale clinical trial. Thus far, none has been done.

Minocycline

As of this writing, a small scale clinical trial of minocycline is underway in Calgary, Canada. Minocycline inhibits aspects of the inflammatory response and seems to have neuroprotective effects in animals.

One reason why promising drugs such as TRH are not tested in large scale, multicenter clinical trials is that they are no longer under a patent, and are therefore not profitable enough for drug companies to do the studies. Such drugs need to be tested with the support of federal research grants. However, government support on such a large scale is difficult to obtain in the U.S., which is why so often these "orphan" drugs are tested in other countries like France. The use of the term "orphan" drugs is not strictly accurate. Orphan drugs are actually drugs that, although useful, are not produced commercially because they are not profitable. Often this is because the patent has run out, but sometimes it is because they are too expensive to manufacture.

Inhibitors of Calcium Entry into Neurons

Nimodipine

In a relatively small French study of 100 patients, the effectiveness of a calcium channel blocker, nimodipine, was tested with and without methylprednisolone and compared to methylprednisolone alone or placebo. Neither nimodipine nor methylprednislone, nor the combination was associated with better outcomes than placebo. Thus, despite the evidence in animal studies that calcium entering injured neurons triggers some of the toxic reactions leading to cell death, inhibitors of the membrane channels that normally regulate entry of calcium into the cell have not proved effective in human SCI—as it also did not prove protective in human stroke.

Small studies such as this one are not conclusive, but neither drug companies nor the federal government are likely to spend huge sums of money to do large scale studies unless preliminary smaller studies suggest that the results will be positive.

Glutamate and Gacyclidine

Another way that calcium enters neurons is through activation of NMDA receptors by the neurotransmitter *glutamate*. It is believed that injured neurons release excessive amounts of glutamate, which binds to the NMDA receptors. These receptors open membrane channels for calcium entry. Thus, administering an inhibitor of NMDA receptors has been neuroprotective in experimental animal models of SCI, traumatic brain injury, and stroke. But, unfortunately, a relatively large study of over 270 patients in 31 hospitals in France failed to show efficacy of intravenous injections of the NMDA receptor inhibitor *gacyclidine*.

Thus far, no method of limiting calcium entry into stretched axons has been devised. Clinical trials of the calcium channel blocker nimodipine and the NMDA receptor blocker gacyclidine did not show improved outcomes and presumably these strategies did not limit calcium-mediated axon disruption.

Surgical Decompression

Spinal cord injury can involve actual penetration of the spinal canal by a missile or bone fragments. This can present a threat to the remaining spinal cord, and surgery might be warranted. As previously discussed, usually the spinal canal is not penetrated, but rather damaged by contusion, which leads to delayed swelling. If the cord swells too much, it becomes too wide for the central canal and could be further damaged by being pressed against the bone. Thus, it is reasonable to suppose that it would be neuroprotective to decompress the cord by removing the overlying bone. However, several studies had failed to document effectiveness of routine surgical decompression compared to medical treatment alone. However, a recent large multicenter trial that compared decompression within the first 24 hours of injury with decompression after 48 hours, suggests a significant benefit for early decompression.

Inhibition of Apoptosis

Even though several strategies to inhibit apoptosis have shown beneficial effects in animal models of stroke, traumatic brain injury, and SCI, convenient drugs to block apoptosis are still not available and no clinical trials have been performed on people with SCI. Given the evidence that SCI includes apoptotic cell death of neurons, microglia, and *oligo-*

dendrocytes (the cells that make myelin in the central nervous system), it seems likely that drugs targeting apoptosis will be developed and subjected to clinical trials.

SUMMARY

Several approaches to neuroprotection have been subjected to randomized clinical trials. However, so far, only methylprednisolone has been proven to be effective. As of this writing, this treatment is being reconsidered; but, intravenous administration of methylprednisolone immediately after SCI is still accepted as the standard of care.

Intravenous administration of methylprednisolone immediately after SCI still accepted as the standard of care.

CHAPTER 9

Research on Repairing the Injured Spinal Cord

A S DISCUSSED IN PREVIOUS CHAPTERS, SCI caused by a concussion results in an expanding area of hemorrhage and cell death, leading to central cord syndrome. The outermost fibers of the descending motor and ascending sensory nerve tracts, which supply motor control and sensation to the lowest segments of the spinal cord, are the most likely to remain undamaged.

Figure 9-1 illustrates some of the ways in which SCI-induced damage to cells can cause loss of neurologic function. Notice that an incomplete concussive injury does not interrupt all the axons. However, some of the axons that are not physically interrupted are nevertheless unable to conduct nerve impulses. They are functionally useless. The reason for this is that SCI causes apoptotic cell death of oligodendrocytes, the cells that make myelin in the central nervous system. When one oligodendrocyte dies, it can cause loss of myelin for as many as forty axons, resulting in blockage of electrical impulses in these axons.

When an axon is severed, the part that is separated from the cell body dies. This is called *Wallerian degeneration*, after the 19th century English doctor and physiologist Augustus Volney Waller. Even if the neuron survives, its neurologic function is lost because its axon no longer communicates with the target neurons in the spinal cord on the other side of the lesion. Injury to an axon also results in retraction of that axon for a short distance just in front of the injury. If the axon had branches that emanated in the portion that was affected by retraction, those branches might also degenerate and lose their function. Even the nerve cell body belonging to the severed axon can undergo degenerative changes, either atrophy (shrinkage) or, in the worst case, cell death. It is believed that this is caused by an interruption of transport of neurotrophic factors from the target regions of the axon backwards to the cell body and nucleus. If the neuron dies, its contribution to neurologic function is permanently lost.

Although it might be possible to limit the loss of neurons and the interruption of axons through neuroprotection strategies, there will

> When an axon is severed, the part that is separated from the cell body dies.

always be a certain degree of damage that is not preventable. In these cases, methods will have to be developed to replace lost neurons, regenerate interrupted axons, and *remyelinate* demyelinated axons. The regenerated axons would also have to be remyelinated.

PROMOTING AXON REGENERATION

Since most loss of function after SCI is due to interruption of axons, with resulting paralysis and loss of sensation below the level of injury, the most urgent need is learn how to encourage regeneration of severed axons. In order to accomplish this, researchers must understand the reasons why axons in the spinal cord do not regenerate by themselves. After all, the axons in peripheral nerves can regenerate, and the axons in the spinal cord of a developing embryo must elongate in order to form the major nerve pathways. So why are axons in the mature central nervous system unable to regrow and reestablish the connections that are needed to restore lost function after SCI?

Collateral Sprouting and Axon Regeneration

Severed axons attempt to regrow when they are interrupted, both in the peripheral nerves and in the central nervous system. This is successful in peripheral nerves, but not in the central nervous system. However, in

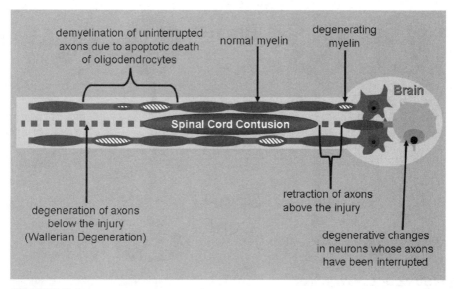

FIGURE 9-1

How SCI Causes Loss of Neurologic Function. This figure illustrates the various types of cellular damage that can result from SCI and contribute to loss of neurologic function. A spinal cord concussive injury produces a contusion (bleeding and cell damage) in the center of the spinal cord at the level of the injury. This can interrupt some axons, resulting in degeneration of the part of the axon that is separated from the cell body by the injury (Wallerian degeneration). This prevents nerve impulses generated by the neuron from being transmitted to target cells in the spinal cord below the injury. The axon also retracts for a short distance above the injury. It is from this point that it would have to regenerate if it were to become functional once more. Some axons that were not severed would also become non-functioning because of the degeneration of the myelin that surrounds them, a consequence of the death of oligodendrocytes. The interruption of an axon can cause a degenerative reaction, sometimes even death, in the neuron cell body. Thus, SCI can cause death of neurons remote from the site of injury, with a total and irreversible loss of their contribution to neurologic function. SCI can also cause death of neurons in the region of injury (not shown). In the case of motor neurons of the cervical and lumbar spinal segments, this could lead to a lower motor neuron syndrome with weakness and atrophy of muscles of the arms and legs.

both locations, neighboring unsevered axons respond to the loss of nearby axons by sending out short sprouts (collateral sprouting) that partially compensate for the degeneration of the injured axons (Figure 9-2).

Collateral sprouting operates over short distances, generally less than 1–2 millimeters. When SCI is incomplete and some axons are spared, collateral sprouting can serve to strengthen the remaining con-

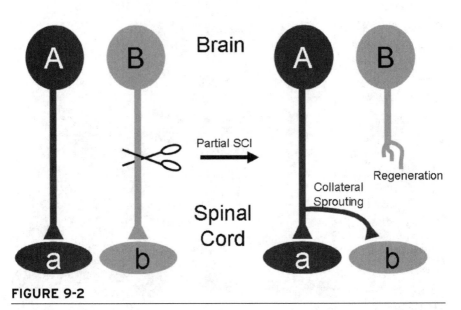

FIGURE 9-2

Collateral sprouting can compensate partially for interrupted axons in SCI. In this diagram, two brain neurons (representing thousands in real life), **A** and **B**, have axons that make synaptic connections with neighboring spinal cord neurons **a** and **b**, respectively. If the axon of neuron **B** is interrupted by a partial SCI (indicated in this cartoon by the scissors) its target cell, neuron **b** loses synaptic input from the brain. The axon of neuron **B** attempts to regenerate, but in the spinal cord this is very limited. However, the axon of neuron **A** sprouts a collateral branch near its terminal and replaces the synapse on neuron **b** that formerly had been made by neuron **B**. Now when neuron **A** is active it activates both neuron **a** and neuron **b**. Although this can compensate partially for the interruption of axon **B**, the patient has lost some of the fine control that previously was enabled by the ability to activate neurons **a** and **b** independently. This loss translates into worsened fine motor skills and other neurologic functions.

nections between the brain and spinal cord, and might account for some of the recovery that ordinarily occurs. Similarly, axons in sensory pathways from the spinal cord can sprout collaterals in the brain, partially compensating for lost sensory axons after SCI.

Because fewer brain neurons are now controlling the activities of the spinal cord neurons, and fewer sensory axons are communicating with the brain, there is inevitably a reduction in fine motor control and sensory discrimination, but the patient might be able to perform many important self care functions and sometimes even walk. However, in the case of anatomically complete SCI where all axons have been severed,

> Severed axons attempt to regrow when they are interrupted, both in the peripheral nerves and in the central nervous system. This is successful in peripheral nerves, but not in the central nervous system.

collateral sprouting could not strengthen the connections between the brain and the spinal cord below the injury. This, in part, accounts for the poor degree of recovery from complete SCI.

Little is known about whether collateral sprouting and regeneration have the same molecular mechanisms. Most of what we do know about the mechanisms of axon elongation comes from the study of embryonic neurons grown in tissue culture. There is a complex structure called a *growth cone* (Figure 9-3) at the tips of their axons, which sends out thin feelers called *filopodia* that taste the environment, stick to an environment they like, and pull the axon along the desired path.

Many of the explanations for the effectiveness of various treatments to enhance regeneration are based on observed effects of drugs on the growth cone, and on the elongation of axons belonging to embryonic neurons in tissue culture. Because these neurons are immature, the mechanisms of axon growth are probably similar to axon elongation during the development of the embryonic nervous system. However, these mechanisms might not be the same as those underlying regeneration of mature, injured axons.

Spinal Cord Molecules that Inhibit Axon Regeneration

In the 1980s, Dr. Albert Aguayo and his collaborators at McGill University discovered that axons in an injured spinal cord can grow for long distances if they are given grafts of peripheral nerve to grow into. This led scientists to conclude that the main problem preventing regeneration of injured axons in the spinal cord was the cellular and molecular environment within the mature central nervous system, rather than an intrinsic inability of mature axons to regenerate.

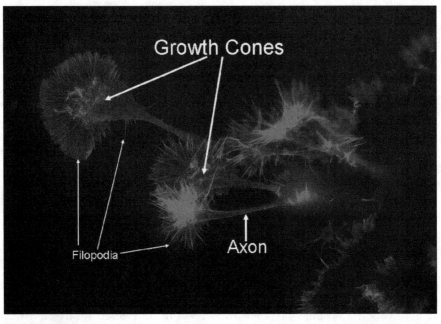

FIGURE 9-3

Growth Cones are the Specialized Endings of Axons Growing in Embryonic Neurons. This is a photomicrograph of axons belonging to embryonic sensory neurons of a chick growing in tissue culture. The neurons are stained with a fluorescently labeled antibody that recognizes actin, the main constituent of the growth cone skeleton. The growth cones are recognizable as complex broadenings at the ends of the axons. The fine tentacle-like projections emanating from the growth cones are called *filopodia*. They sense the chemical environment of the axon, participate in pulling it along and help steer it as it grows. It is still not clear to what degree growth cones are responsible for pulling mature injured axons during regeneration.

This conclusion was probably premature, because only a small fraction of the injured axons regenerated into the nerve grafts, and other evidence suggests that, with maturity, neurons lose much of their intrinsic ability to regenerate. This means that in order to obtain sufficient regeneration to restore function, both the environmental factors and the intrinsic maturational changes that retard axon regeneration in the spinal cord will have to be overcome.

Some surgeons have attempted to bridge a spinal cord injury with grafts of peripheral nerve, but there is little evidence of therapeutic benefit, perhaps because only a few axons regenerate, but more importantly, perhaps also because once the regenerated axons reach the end of the graft, their ability to grow back into the spinal cord on the other side is still very limited. In any case, these attempts have not been published in peer-reviewed journal articles and have not been part of controlled clinical trials, making it difficult to interpret the results if an occasional patient improved.

Hundreds of people with SCI have received transplants of a type of glial cell called *olfactory ensheathing cells* (OEC), primarily in China. The rationale for this treatment is that the sensory neurons of the nerve fibers that transmit information about odors from the nose to the brain are constantly dying and regenerating. Thus, axons are constantly regenerating from the nose to the brain. It was speculated that the glial cells that surround these axons must be especially supportive of regeneration. Some experiments using animals suggested that transplanting these cells into a partial spinal cord injury could enhance regeneration and promote functional recovery. Not all scientists agreed with this conclusion, but the news was so exciting that the medical community and many people with SCI were convinced to have the procedure done. Once again, there was little evidence that the therapy is helpful. No controlled clinical trials were performed, and results were not published in peer-reviewed journals. A very small Phase I clinical trial of OEC transplantation is underway in Australia.

Nogo and Other Molecules in Myelin that Inhibit Regeneration

With Dr. Aguayo's discoveries in mind, the search began to find molecules in the central nervous system that blocked axon regeneration. In Switzerland, scientists discovered a protein present in the myelin of central nervous system axons that caused the tips of axons growing in tissue culture to collapse and stop elongating. The molecule was absent from myelin in peripheral nerve, which actually promotes axon regeneration. Eventually, the amino acid sequence of the molecule was determined, and the molecule was given the humorous name *Nogo* by the doctor who discovered it: Dr. Martin Schwab.

Nogo acts by binding to a receptor molecule embedded in the membrane of the growth cone (Figure 9-4). The Nogo receptor forms a complex with two other receptor molecules. When Nogo binds to its receptor, it triggers a cascade of biochemical reactions that causes the filopodia of the growth cone to retract, the growth cone itself to collapse, and the axon to stop growing. An antibody to Nogo was found to enhance collateral sprouting, and possibly even axon regeneration in animals subjected to partial spinal cord injury. These animals also showed more behavioral recovery than animals treated with control antibodies.

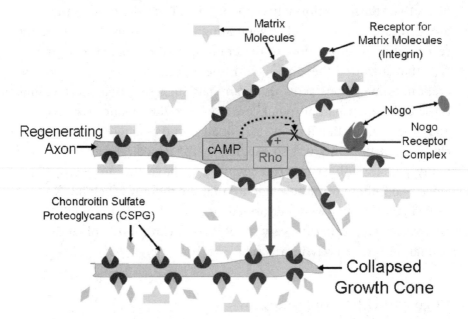

FIGURE 9-4

Molecules Can Inhibit Axon Growth by Different Mechanisms. This figure illustrates an axon with a broad growth cone at its tip. Filopodia emanating from the growth cone help guide and pull the axon forward. Embedded in the growth cone membrane are receptors for many molecules, including Nogo. When Nogo binds to its receptor, it triggers a cascade of biochemical signals that causes the growth cone to collapse and the axon to stop growing. An important part of that cascade of biochemical signals is activation of an enzyme called *Rho*. A growth-promoting signal, cyclic AMP (cAMP) blocks activation of Rho and prevents growth cone collapse. Not all regeneration-blocking molecules cause growth cone collapse. Chondroitin sulfate proteoglycans (CSPG) are molecules that are made by glial cells at the site of a SCI. CSPG block axon growth by binding to the receptors (called *integrins*) in the cell membrane that allow the cell to stick to the extracellular matrix.

Therefore, the pharmaceutical company Novartis performed a Phase I open label (not controlled, not blinded) clinical trial in Europe, involving injection of the antibody (ATI-355) into the spinal fluid soon after injury. Patients with complete SCI (ASIA A) were selected because researchers felt these patients had less to lose than people with partial injury, in case the treatment had serious toxic side effects. So far, the drug has not caused major toxicity, and as of this writing a Phase II trial is being planned for North America.

Other molecules found in central nervous system myelin also have been shown to inhibit axon growth. Among them, *myelin-associated glycoprotein* (MAG) and *oligodendrocyte myelin glycoprotein* (OMGP; MOG) are also growth cone collapsing molecules. Interestingly, they both bind to the Nogo receptor and inhibit axon growth by triggering the same cascade of intracellular events as Nogo, even though they are very different from Nogo in their chemical makeup. This means that even if you eliminated Nogo, it is possible that the same growth cone collapsing effects would occur because of the redundancy of the inhibitory signaling. Therefore, some scientists have been experimenting with a more general approach that would neutralize all three molecules that bind to the Nogo receptor. This has not yet advanced to the point of clinical trials.

Rho and Cyclic AMP

The intracellular molecular signaling cascade that links Nogo binding to its receptor with collapse of the growth cone involves activation of an enzyme called *Rho* (Figure 9-4). Studies using animals have suggested the drugs that inhibit Rho can enhance axon sprouting or regeneration in models of partial SCI and help increase functional recovery. BioAxone Therapeutic initiated an open label clinical trial of Cethrine (BA-210; licensed to Alseres Pharmaceuticals), an inhibitor of Rho that is applied to the surface of the thick membrane (*dura mater*) that surrounds the spinal cord.

As with anti-Nogo antibody treatment, patients with complete SCI were selected because they have less to lose than people with partial injury. After completion of Phase I/IIa, the drug appeared to have little toxicity. Therefore, the company has teamed up with a larger company, Boston Life Sciences, Alseres Pharmaceuticals is planning to perform a Phase II clinical trial.

The molecule *cyclic AMP* (cAMP) is a common intracellular signal that has many effects on neurons. One of its effects is inhibition of Rho activation (Figure 8-4). Therefore, one effect of cAMP is to block the growth cone collapsing activity of Nogo and other growth cone collapsing molecules. In animals, administration of drugs that increase the activity of cAMP within cells, increased axon sprouting or regeneration, and enhanced functional recovery in models of partial SCI, especially when combined with additional strategies, such as transplantation of Schwann cells (see below). Although cAMP-like drugs have been tested in clinical trials for other diseases, as of this writing, no clinical trial of a cAMP-like drug has been initiated for SCI.

Chondroitin Sulfate Proteoglycans

In order for an axon to grow, it must adhere to surrounding tissue. This is accomplished because the extracellular environment through which the axon grows contains molecules that form a sticky matrix. The neuron cell membrane contains receptor molecules called *integrins* to which these extracellular matrix molecules bind, triggering a series of intracellular events leading to axon growth.

At the site of SCI, the glial cells secrete several molecules that influence axon regeneration, some promoting it and some inhibiting it. One family of molecules that are secreted by the injured glial cells, and that

> In order for an axon to grow, it must adhere to surrounding tissue.

are inhibitory to axon growth, is the chondroitin sulfate proteoglycans (CSPG). These molecules bind to the same site on the integrins as the matrix molecules (Figure 9-4). This inhibits the growing axon from adhering properly to the surrounding tissue and blocks the axon from growing. Application of an enzyme (chondroitinase ABC) that digests (breaks down) the CSPG was shown to enhance axon sprouting or regeneration in animal models of spinal cord injury and improved functional recovery. Although clinical trials are in the planning stage, none have been initiated as of this writing.

Cytokines and Neurotrophic Factors

We have already been introduced to neurotrophic factors: the small proteins that are secreted by target cells and are required by the neuron in very small quantities to maintain health and sometimes even its very survival. When certain trophic factors were applied directly to the injured spinal cords of rats with partial SCI, or when cells genetically engineered to make trophic factors were transplanted into their injured spinal cords, axon sprouting and/or regeneration was enhanced and functional recovery increased. Although transplantation of these neurotrophin-secreting cells into the brain is currently undergoing clinical trials in patients with Alzheimer's disease, there are no clinical trials of neurotrophic factors yet for SCI.

Neurotrophic factors can be thought of as a specific form of a larger class of molecules (cytokines). These are proteins that are secreted by cells into the extracellular environment, bind to specific receptors on the surfaces of the same or different cells, and activate intracellular biochemical signaling pathways that serve many functions. Like neurotrophic factors, some cytokines promote growth and regeneration of neurons, but some cytokines can actually be toxic to neurons and/or inhibitory to axon regeneration.

Many cytokines are secreted by immunological cells, and this has given rise to attempts to manipulate the immunological system in such a way as to promote axon regeneration. For example, it was found that certain immunological cells (macrophages) change the types of cytokines and neurotrophins that they secrete when they are activated by coming in contact with a foreign body. Macrophages are white blood cells that detect foreign bodies, ingest them by phagocytosis, and then digest them.

Rat macrophages that were activated by incubating them with skin or nerve tissue secreted more of some neurotrophic factors and cytokines that promote axon regeneration and less of some cytokines that inhibit regeneration.

Experiments using rats also suggested that intraspinal injection of activated macrophages were neuroprotective and resulted in enhanced recovery after SCI, although evidence for regeneration was sketchy. On the strength of these animal studies, Proneuron Biotechnologies undertook clinical trials in which patients' own macrophages were activated by incubating them with pieces of the patients' own skin, and then injected into their spinal cords near the injury site. These were patients who had suffered a complete (ASIA A) cervical or thoracic SCI. Phase I was completed in Israel and Belgium, and did not suggest major toxicity. A Phase II trial was then initiated in the U.S., but it has been suspended for lack of funds.

Remyelinating Axons

Axons that have lost myelin as a result of SCI, and axons that have been induced to regenerate, must be remyelinated. Scientists have created precursors of oligodendrocytes, and have injected them into the spinal cords of rats. They have shown that these cells can mature into oligodendrocytes and make myelin. So far, no clinical trial has been performed on humans, but as of this writing one is being planned.

Another idea for remyelinating axons is to inject Schwann cells into the spinal cord. Schwann cells are the cells that make myelin in peripheral nerves. Schwann cells can remyelinate spinal cord axons in experimental animals. They are thought to produce neurotrophic factors and other molecules that promote regeneration of axons in peripheral nerve, and their injection into the spinal cord might have the additional advantage that they would promote regeneration of interrupted axons as well as remyelinating them. To date, no clinical trials have been performed, but many patients have received Schwann cell transplants in China. Although improvement has been claimed, results have not been published in peer reviewed journals.

REPLACING LOST NEURONS

Neurons that have died as a result of SCI cannot regenerate by themselves. They would have to be replaced in order to recover lost functioning. An example would be the motor neurons of the cervical spinal cord in the case of a C5–6 SCI. If these motor neurons die, the muscles they innervate in the shoulder and arm will become paralyzed and atro-

> Neurons that have died as a result of SCI cannot regenerate by themselves.

phy. Ideally, the motor neurons would have to be replaced soon enough to prevent the muscles from becoming so atrophied that they cannot be brought back to health by reinnervation.

Neural Stem Cells

Many people have heard that the brain and spinal cord have neural stem cells that are always dividing and have the potential, through a process of progressive specialization, to become any of the neural cell types, including neurons, *astrocytes* (also called *astroglia*, non-neuronal supporting glial cells in the central nervous system) and oligodendrocytes (also called *oligodendroglia*, the specialized glial cells that make myelin in the central nervous system).

Stem cells are constantly dividing and forming one of two types of cell. Either they form two daughter stem cells, similar to themselves, or they form cells that are one step more specialized (Figure 9-5). For example a neural stem cell might divide and one of the daughter cells might become a neuronal precursor cell—a cell that is now committed to becoming a neuron. Alternatively, a neural stem cell might continue to divide, producing more neuronal precursors, some of which might then become precursors of more specific neuron types, such as motor neurons. This means that the cell could continue to divide or differentiate into a motor neuron, but it could not become an astrocyte or even a

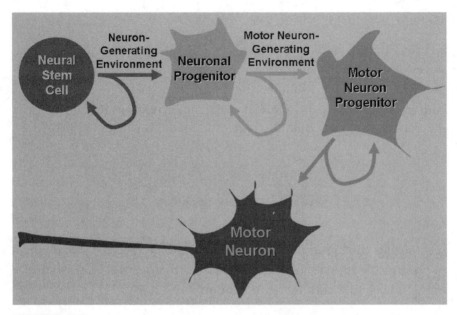

FIGURE 9-5

Neural Stem Cells Can Become Specific Neuron Types Through a Process of Progressive Differentiation. This is a simplified representation of the general process by which stem cells are thought to become differentiated neurons, using the motor neuron as an example. The actual number of steps is probably greater than illustrated. Stem cells and progenitor cells are capable of dividing and regenerating themselves indefinitely. However, under correct conditions, they can undergo partial differentiation and become committed to a particular type of tissue or cell type. Neural stem cells are not true pleuripotent stem cells because they are not able to become any cell type in the body. Instead, they have already acquired a commitment to become cells of the nervous system. However, they can become any neural cell type—neuron, astrocyte or oligodendrocyte. In an environment that has the correct mix of neurotrophic factors and other molecules, neural stem cells can be coaxed to commit to a neuron-generating cell line; for example, they can become neuronal progenitors. These cells can still divide and regenerate themselves, but under the correct conditions, they can further differentiate into progenitors of specific types of neurons, such as motor neurons. Finally, the motor neuron progenitor can stop dividing and become a differentiated motor neuron. Each step is normally irreversible.

different type of neuron. In the case of neurons, this terminal differentiation renders the cells incapable of further cell division.

Under normal conditions, each step in this process of progressive differentiation is irreversible, although some scientists have been able to reverse the process to a limited extent and under very artificial conditions. Recently, scientists may have even made pleuripotent embryonic stem cells out of adult skin cells. Whether stem cells become more differentiated and, if so, in which direction, is influenced by chemicals in their environment, especially neurotrophic factors and related molecules. Neuroscientists have learned a great deal about how to drive the differentiation in selected ways so they can generate neurons from stem cells in a tissue culture dish by exposing the cells to the correct mix of neurotrophic factors and other molecules.

Why the Spinal Cord Cannot Generate New Neurons

New neurons are constantly being made in some parts of the adult brain. However, this is not true in the spinal cord, even though the spinal cord has neural stem cells. These same cells can be removed from the cord and induced to become neurons in tissue culture. So why doesn't the spinal cord respond to injury by just making more neurons to replace the ones that have died? As stated above, stem cells are influenced by chemicals in their environment, especially neurotrophic factors and related molecules. For some reason having to do with the types of neurotrophic factors and other molecules expressed by cells in the spinal cord, stem cells in the cord can become glial cells but not neurons. This is also true of stem cells derived from brain tissue and transplanted into the spinal cord. Clearly, the environment of the spinal cord is not conducive to the generation of neurons, and injecting neural stem cells into an injured spinal cord will not give rise to more neurons.

Neuronal Progenitors

Neuroscientists have learned a great deal about how to promote the differentiation of stem cells in selected ways, so they can generate neurons from stem cells in a tissue culture dish by exposing the cells to the correct mix of neurotrophic factors and other molecules. When stem cells are induced to become neuronal progenitors in this way, they can then be transplanted into the spinal cord of experimental animals and, because they are committed to a neuronal fate, they can become neurons.

Until now, this possibility has not been developed to the point of potential clinical usefulness, but several laboratories are working on it. It is interesting that many people with SCI have received transplants of stem cells derived from bone marrow or from human embryonic brain in China and elsewhere. These procedures were not part of a randomized controlled prospective clinical trial, or even any kind of controlled trial. The results have not been published in peer reviewed research articles, and there is no good evidence that the patients benefited. We do not know what became of these transplanted cells, but given all the experimental evidence in animals, it is very unlikely that they became neurons.

SUMMARY

SCI involves several types of damage to nerve cells, including death of neurons near to and remote from the injury, not only because of direct consequences of the impact but also because of delayed cell death, loss of myelin in axons near to and remote from the injury, and interruption of axons that carry signals between the brain and spinal cord. Rapid progress in the area of stem cell biology, and the results of animal experiments, have given rise to hopes that some day we may be able to replace lost neurons and myelin, but although surgeons in some countries have been transplanting stem cells into human SCI patients, there is as yet no published evidence for clinical benefit, and so far no prospective controlled clinical trials have been undertaken. To some degree, the more critical problem is the failure of injured axons to regenerate after they have been interrupted. Scientists have learned a great deal about the reasons for this failure of regeneration. These include the existence of inhibitory molecules in the environment of the axon, as well as age-related changes in the intrinsic regenerative capacity of neurons that develop after birth. Although here too, progress has been made in experimental animals, clinical trials aimed at promoting axon regeneration in human SCI patients are still in early phases (Phase I). However, some Phase I studies have been completed and Phase II trials are planned. Within a very few years, we should know whether the optimism based on animal experiments is justified.

Internet Resources for Spinal Cord Injury

ABLEDATA (for products and consumer guides): www.abledata.com

American Academy of Neurology (AAN): www.aan.com

American Academy of Physical Medicine and Rehabilitation (AAPM&R): www.aapmr.org

American Congress of Rehabilitation Medicine (ACRM): www.acrm.org

American Society of NeuroRehabilitation (ASNR): www.asnr.com

American Spinal Injury Association (ASIA; primarily for doctors and researchers):

www.asia-spinalinjury.org

Christopher Reeve Paralysis Foundation Paralysis Resource Center: www.paralysis.org

Disabled Dealer Magazine (for modified vehicles): www.disableddealer.com

Eastern Paralyzed Veterans of America United Spinal Association: www.unitedspinal.org

International Campaign for Cures of Spinal Cord Injury Paralysis (ICCP): www.campaignforcure.org

National Center for Medical Rehabilitation Research (NCMRR; a branch of the National Institute of Child health and Human Development): www.nichd.nih.gov/about/org/ncmrr

National Institute on Disability and Rehabilitation Research (NIDRR, a branch of the US Department of Education): www.ed.gov/about/offices/list/osers/nidrr/index.html

National Institutes of Health (NIH) information about stem cells: http://stemcells.nih.gov/info/faqs.asp

National Institute of Neurologic Diseases and Stroke: www.ninds.nih.gov

National Multiple Sclerosis Society: www.nationalmssociety.org

National Organization on Disability (for disability rights): www.nod.org

New Mobility (lifestyles for people in wheelchairs): www.newmobility.com

Paralyzed Veterans of America (for advocacy, technology, updates on research): www.pva.org

SCI Model Systems Program for SCI data: www.spinalcord.uab.edu

Veterans Health Administration: http://www1.va.gov/health/aboutvha.asp

Glossary

TERMS USED IN THIS BOOK or in other sources of information about SCI. Adapted with permission from the Paralysis Resource Guide, by Sam Maddox, The Christopher and Dana Reeve Paralysis Resource Center.

4-Aminopyridine (4-AP)—an experimental drug currently in clinical trials for MS and spinal cord injury that improves conduction of nerve impulses; can cause seizure, convulsion, or dizziness.

Abdominal binder—a wide elastic binder used to help prevent hypotension (drop in blood pressure) or used for cosmetic purposes to hold in abdomen.

Acute—a stage of injury or stroke starting at the onset of symptoms; the opposite of chronic.

ADL—rehabilitation shorthand for "activities of daily living," such as dressing, eating, cooking.

Amyotrophic Lateral Sclerosis (ALS)—a disorder involving loss of use of muscles. The nerve cells controlling these muscles (motor neurons) are destroyed; also known as Lou Gehrig's disease.

Anoxia—a state of almost no oxygen delivery to a cell, resulting in low energy production and possible death of the cell.

Anticoagulants—a drug therapy used to prevent the formation of blood clots that can become lodged in cerebral arteries and cause strokes.

Anticholinergic—a type of drug often prescribed to reduce spasms of smooth muscle, including the bladder; opposes the actions of the neurotransmitter acetylcholine.

Antiplatelet agents—a type of anticoagulant drug therapy that prevents the formation of blood clots by preventing the accumulation of platelets that form the basis of blood clots; some common antiplatelet drugs include aspirin, clopidogrel and ticlopidine; see anticoagulants.

Aphasia—the inability to understand or create speech, writing, or language; generally due to damage to the speech centers of the brain.

Apoptosis—a form of cell suicide that does not induce an inflammatory response, often called programmed cell death because it is triggered by a genetic signal, involves specific cell mechanisms, and is irreversible once initiated.

Arteriovenous malformation (AVM)—a congenital disorder characterized by a complex tangled web of arteries and veins.

ASIA Score—a measure of function after spinal cord injury, used by doctors, in which dysfunction is graded from A–E. A means complete injury; E means full recovery.

Astrocyte—a star-shaped glial support cell that helps provide the chemical environment for nerve regeneration, but also secretes molecules that block regeneration.

Ataxia—loss of balance; a problem of movement coordination not due to weakness, rigidity, or spasticity.

Atelectasis—the collapse of part or all of a lung by blockage of the air passages, or by shallow breathing.

Atherosclerosis—a blood vessel disease characterized by deposits of lipid material on the inside of the walls of large to medium-sized arteries which make the artery walls thick, hard, brittle, and prone to breaking.

Atrophy—loss of bulk in a muscle, nerve, or an organ, from less than normal usage or from previous damage; can also occur because of lack of needed trophic factors or nutrients.

Autonomic dysreflexia—a potentially dangerous reaction (sweating, chills, high blood pressure) to a stimulus below the level of lesion in people with injuries to the spinal cord above T6; untreated can lead to stroke.

Axon—the nerve fiber or process that carries a nerve impulse from the nerve cell body to the nerve terminals; for sensory neurons, the axon can also carry the nerve impulse from the sensory nerve terminals in the body back to the nerve cell.

Blood-brain barrier—The special property of capillaries in the brain that prevents the passage of large molecules, electrically charged molecules (ions) and many drugs from the blood into the brain or spinal cord; protects neurons from the toxic effects of direct exposure to blood.

Brown-Sequard syndrome—an incomplete spinal cord injury, wherein half of the cord has been damaged. There is spastic paralysis and loss of vibration and joint position sense on the same side as the lesion, and loss of other sensations on the opposite side of the lesion.

Catheter—a rubber or plastic tube used to drain urine from the bladder.

Cauda equina—the spinal roots of the lower lumbar and sacral spinal cord segments descending in the spinal canal below the end of the spinal cord.

Central nervous system (CNS)—nerve tissue within the brain and spinal cord.

Central pain (central pain syndrome)—pain that arises from injury to the central nervous system rather than from bodily injury. It is a mixture of sensations, including heat and cold, burning, tingling, numbness, and sharp stabbing and underlying aching pain.

Cerebrospinal fluid (CSF)—the circulating clear fluid that bathes the brain and spinal cord, protecting it from shock.

Cervical—the portion of the spinal cord in the neck area.

Chondroitin sulfate proteoglycans—a family of chemicals that inhibit axon regeneration; released by astrocytes at the site of an injury.

Chronic—a condition that is continuous or persistent over an extended period of time, not easily or quickly resolved; the opposite of acute.

Clonus—involuntary movement of rapidly alternating contraction and relaxation of a muscle. It is the result of overactive tendon reflexes, reflecting injury to the descending motor pathways from the cerebral cortex to the spinal cord.

Complete injury—generally, a spinal cord injury that cuts off all sensory and motor function below the lesion site.

Computed tomography (CT) scan—a reconstruction of the structure of tissues, such as the brain and head, achieved by using a computer to analyze a series of X-rays taken at different angles; also called computerized axial tomography or CAT scan.

Concussion (a concussive injury)—reversible loss of consciousness and/or a transient state of confusion due to brain trauma.

Contracture—a joint that has stiffened to the point it cannot be moved through its normal range.

Cyclic AMP—an important intracellular signaling molecule that has many functions and enhances axon regeneration.

Cyst—a cavity in the spinal cord that fills with fluid and can lead to loss of function, pain; same as syrinx; see syringomyelia.

Cystogram—an X-ray of the bladder to show reflux (backward flow of urine back to the kidneys).

Cytokines—small, hormone-like proteins secreted by immunological (and sometimes other) cells. Cytokines bind to specific receptors on target cells to activate intracellular signals with varying effects, such as promoting an inflammatory immune response to injury.

Cytotoxic edema—an influx of fluids and toxic chemicals into a cell causing swelling of the cell.

Decubitus—a skin sore cause by unrelieved pressure.

Demyelination—the loss of nerve insulation called myelin, generally leading to loss of nerve function. Common in multiple sclerosis (MS) and spinal cord injury.

Dermatome—the territory of sensation served by the nerve fibers of a given spinal cord segment.

Dysphagia—trouble eating and swallowing.

Edema—the swelling of a cell or tissue from large amounts of water or fluid that have entered the cell or tissue.

Electro-ejaculation—a method of obtaining viable sperm from men who are unable to produce a sample by other means; uses an electrical probe in the rectum.

Embolic stroke—a stroke caused by an embolus, a free-roaming clot that usually forms in the heart.

Exacerbation—in certain diseases (for example, multiple sclerosis) a recurrence or worsening of symptoms.

Excitatory amino acids—a type of neurotransmitter; proteins released at a synapse by one neuron to promote an excitatory state in the other neuron.

Excitotoxicity—damage to nerve and glial cells caused by excessive release of excitatory neurotransmitters, especially glutamate; can also be produced artificially by extrinsic application of the neurotransmitter or a drug that mimics it.

Friedreich's ataxia—an inherited, progressive dysfunction of the cerebellum, spinal cord, and peripheral nerves.

Functional Electrical Stimulation (FES)—application of electrical currents to nerves or paralyzed muscles in order to activate the muscles artificially. Facilitates exercise, ambulation, grip, bladder control, etc.

Functional magnetic resonance imaging (fMRI)—a type of imaging that uses MRI to measure blood flow or oxygen use within the brain during performance of a mental or physical task, thereby demonstrating the anatomic location of areas of the brain involved in performing that task.

Glasgow Coma Scale (GCS)—A rating scale devised by Teasdale and Jennett to assess the level of consciousness following brain damage. The scale assesses eye, verbal and motor responses. The GCS is graded 1–15, the lower score indicating the greater neurologic impairment.

Glia—also called *neuroglia*; supportive (derived from the Greek for glue) cells of the nervous system that surround neural structures and blood vessels, provide nutrients and oxygen to the neurons, and protect the neurons from infection, toxicity, and trauma. There are three kinds of glia: oligodendroglia, astrocytes, and microglia.

Glutamate—glutamic acid, an amino acid that acts as an excitatory neurotransmitter in the brain.

Growth cone—the specialized ending of a growing axon that probes the chemical environment and pulls the axon forward; may be more characteristic of embryonic neurons than regenerating mature axons.

Guillain-Barré syndrome—an acute inflammation of peripheral nerve that damages the myelin (insulation) of the axon, resulting in muscle weakness or paralysis and variably, also numbness.

Hemiparesis—weakness on one side of the body.

Hemiplegia—paralysis on one side of the body.

Hemorrhagic stroke—sudden bleeding into the brain.

Heterotopic ossification—bone deposits in the connective tissues around the hips, knees and other joints, generally due to inactivity.

Hippocampus—a portion of the temporal lobe of the brain that is implicated in memory and learning.

Hydrocephalus—a disorder associated with excessive cerebrospinal fluid in the brain, resulting in abnormal enlargement of the ventricles; accompanies certain types of spinal bifida.

Hyperbaric oxygen therapy—a system of delivering pressurized oxygen to help treat decompression sickness (the bends), smoke inhalation, air embolism, and other conditions.

Hypothermia—a technique to cool the spinal cord or brain after trauma; can reduce swelling and reduce the metabolic requirements of damaged tissue.

Hypoxia—abnormally reduced oxygen delivery to a cell.

Immune response—the body's defense mechanism involving white blood cells and related cells to attack and eliminate microorganisms, viruses, and substances recognized as foreign and potentially harmful.

Incomplete spinal cord injury—a spinal cord injury with preserved sensory or motor function below the lesion level.

Incontinence—loss of control of bowel or bladder.

Indwelling catheter—a flexible tube that remains in the bladder for continuous draining.

Intermittent catheter—a flexible tube that is inserted repeatedly to empty the bladder on a regular schedule; self-catheterization.

Infarct—an area of tissue that is dead or dying because of a loss of blood supply.

Interleukins—a group of cytokines involved in the inflammatory immune response of the ischemic cascade.

Intracerebral hemorrhage—leakage of blood into the brain due to rupture of a brain blood vessel.

Intrathecal—into the cerebrospinal fluid within the arachnoid membrane that surrounds the brain and spinal cord; often used in reference to delivery of drugs (for example, the spasm-controlling drug baclofen, or the pain-killer morphine) by way of a small, implanted pump, allowing for higher dosage applied to the central nervous system than could be tolerated if the drug were administered systemically (by mouth or injected into the bloodstream). Reduces toxic side effects.

Intravenous pyelogram (IVP)—a type of X-ray to study the kidneys, bladder, and ureters (the tubes which carry urine from the kidneys to the bladder) by the intravenous injection of a radio-opaque dye.

Ischemia—a loss of blood flow to tissue, caused by an obstruction of the blood vessel.

Ischemic cascade—a series of events lasting for several hours to several days following initial ischemia that results in extensive cell death and tissue damage beyond the area originally affected by the initial lack of blood flow.

Ischemic stroke—irreversible damage to the brain due to obstructed blood flow.

Laminectomy—an operation to relieve pressure on the spinal cord by chipping away the roof of the spine.

Lesion—the site of injury or wound (to the spinal cord).

Leukocytes—white blood cells; they are involved in the inflammatory immune response of the ischemic cascade.

Lower motor neurons—nerve cells of the spinal cord and brainstem whose axons leave the central nervous system and travel in the peripheral nerves to the muscles. An injury to these nerves can cause muscle weakness and also can affect bowel, bladder and sexual functions.

Lumbar—the thickest section of the spine, below the thoracic area.

Magnetic resonance imaging (MRI)—a type of imaging scan that uses computers to analyze the effects of imposed magnetic fields on the tissues. Can detect subtle changes in the water content and other chemical properties of tissues. Results in high resolution images of brain and spinal cord that are sensitive to strokes and other disorders.

Methylprednisolone—steroid drug given to people with spinal cord trauma within 8 hours of injury; a neuroprotective drug that increases the chances for functional recovery.

Multiple sclerosis (MS)—a chronic disease of the central nervous system characterized by loss of myelin.

Myelin—white, fatty insulating material on axons that helps rapid conduction of nerve impulses. Loss of myelin accompanies MS, spinal cord injury and other neurologic conditions.

Myelomeningocele—a neural tube birth defect, a form of spina bifida usually accompanied by paralysis, wherein a portion of the spinal cord or spinal nerve roots protrudes from the spinal column.

Necrosis—a form of cell death resulting from anoxia, trauma, or any other form of irreversible damage to the cell; involves the release of toxic cellular material into the intercellular space, poisoning surrounding cells.

Neurogenic bladder—a bladder with any disturbance due to an injury of the nervous system.

Neurologist—a doctor who specializes in the medical treatment of diseases and disorders of the brain, spinal cord, nerves and muscles.

Neuron—the primary cell of the nervous system that is responsible for rapid transmission of information by the use of electrical signals; consists of a cell body, an axon, and dendrites.

Neuroprotective agents—medications that protect the brain from secondary injury caused by stroke or trauma; an example is methylprednisolone.

Neurosurgeon—a doctor who specializes in the surgical treatment of diseases and disorders of the brain, spinal cord, and nerves.

NMDA receptor—abbreviated name of the n-methyl-d-aspartate receptor for the neurotransmitter glutamine. This receptor is linked to a pore in the membrane that allows calcium to enter the neuron and is important in many processes of the central nervous system, such as memory and learning. It is also involved in generating some of the delayed damage to neurons following spinal cord injury.

Nogo—a protein found in central nervous system myelin that inhibits axon regeneration.

Oligodendrocyte—the support cell in the central nervous system that makes myelin.

Orthosis—a device applied outside of the body to support the body and limbs or to assist motion.

Ostomy—an opening in the body to drain the bladder (cystostomy), to remove solid waste (colostomy or ileostomy) or allow passage of air (tracheostomy).

Oxygen-free radicals—toxic chemicals produced by the peroxidation of fatty substances in the cell that are released in excessive amounts during necrosis of a cell; involved in secondary cell death associated with the ischemic cascade.

PCA—personal care attendant.

Paraplegia—paralysis and other loss of function below the cervical area; generally, upper body, including arms, retains motor and sensory function.

Passive standing—use of a frame or device to stand a person who cannot do so otherwise; has benefits for bone strength.

Peripheral nervous system—nerves in the body away from the brain and spinal cord; have ability for self-repair that the central system axons do not.

Physiatrist—a doctor who specializes in physical medicine and rehabilitation.

Plasticity—the ability to be formed or molded; in reference to the brain, the ability to adapt to changed patterns of use and disuse, including those due to disease and injury.

Poliomyelitis (polio)—a viral disease of the central nervous system that attacks the motor neurons. It is transmitted only by humans, leaves the body within a few months of infection, but often leaves people with weakened or paralyzed limbs. Outside research labs, no polio has been found in the U.S. for over 20 years, but polio still exists in some parts of the world. Pressure sore—a skin breakdown due to unrelieved pressure.

Quadriplegia—also known as *tetraplegia*; paralysis affecting all four limbs.

Range of motion—normal movement of a joint.

Reflux—the flow of urine backwards into the kidneys; can lead to kidney breakdown.

Regeneration—the regrowth and reconnection of nerves. Occurs routinely in the peripheral nervous system. Can be induced experimentally in brain or spinal cord experiments but functional regeneration in human SCI patients faces many hurdles.

Retrograde pyelogram (RP)—a tool to diagnose kidney function using contrast material injected into the urethra and bladder.

Rhizotomy—the cutting of spinal or cranial (brain) nerve roots to interrupt spasticity or pain signals.

Rho—an enzyme that is part of the intracellular signaling involved in the regeneration-blocking effect of Nogo and other growth cone collapsing molecules.

Spasticity—uncontrolled increase in muscle tone; muscle stiffness resulting from continuous activity or from overactive stretch reflexes. Can be beneficial by helping legs to support the body's weight, but can also interfere with daily activities.

Spinal shock—after spinal trauma, a condidtion similar to a coma from brain concussion; the nervous system shuts down, with loss of reflexes in the limbs, and the body becomes flaccid. Can last three or four weeks.

Stroke—a "brain attack" or sudden loss of neurological function caused by death of brain tissue due to blockage of a blood vessel (or bleeding in the case of hemorrhagic stroke). The word "stroke" implies a sudden event. However, occasionally the symptoms of a stroke can build up over several hours or even days, giving rise to misdiagnosis as brain tumor or abscess.

Subarachnoid hemorrhage—bleeding within the meninges, the outer membranes of the brain, into the clear fluid that surrounds the brain.

Suprapubic cystostomy—an opening through the abdomen to drain the bladder with a catheter; known as a "super tube."

Syringomyelia—a disorder caused by formation of a fluid-filled cavity within the spinal cord. Frequently occurs after SCI.

Tendonesis—a hand splint made of metal or plastic, used to increase hand function.

Tendon transfer—a type of hand surgery that offers qualified quadriplegics significant increase in hand function. Takes advantage of functioning muscles in the arms by moving the tendons that control the hands.

Tethered cord—occurs when scar tissue develops between the lower end of the spinal cord and the dura mater or arachnoid, two of the membranes covering the spinal cord and brain. Tethering is believed to create and/or worsen symptoms of an existing syrinx. If symptomatic, surgeons can meticulously untether a cord.

Thoracic—the portion of the spinal column in the chest, between the cervical and lumbar areas.

Thrombolytics—drugs used to treat an ongoing, acute ischemic stroke by dissolving the blood clot causing the stroke, thereby restoring blood flow through the artery.

Tissue necrosis factors—chemicals released by leukocytes and other cells that cause secondary cell death during the inflammatory immune response associated with the ischemic cascade.

Transverse myelitis—inflammation in the spinal cord interfering with nerve function below the level of the inflammation; an acute attack of inflammatory demyelination.

Upper motor neurons—these are the nerve cells that originate in the brain whose long axons travel through the spinal cord. Disruption of these cells leads to paralysis although some reflex activity is still possible.

Warfarin—a commonly used anticoagulant, also known as Coumadin®.

Index

NOTE: Boldface numbers indicate illustrations; italic *t* indicates a table.